The Best of Friends

Two Sisters, One Journey

Connie Kiosse

Copyright © 2003 by Connie Kiosse

ISBN 0-7414-1739-1

Published by:

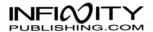
PUBLISHING.COM

519 West Lancaster Avenue
Haverford, PA 19041-1413
Info@buybooksontheweb.com
www.buybooksontheweb.com
Toll-free (877) BUY BOOK
Local Phone (610) 520-2500
Fax (610) 519-0261

Printed in the United States of America

Printed on Recycled Paper

Published October 2003

For my sister, Christine

I am standing on the seashore. A ship at my side spreads her white sails to the morning breeze and starts for the blue ocean. She is an object of beauty and strength. I stand and watch her until at length she is only a ribbon of white cloud just where the sea and sky come to mingle with each other. There! She is gone! But someone at my side says, "Gone Where?" From our sight that is all. She is just as large in mast and hull and spar as when she left our side, and just as able to bear her load of living freight to the place of destination. Her diminished size is in us, not her. Just at the moment when you say, "There! She is gone!" other voices are ready to take up the glad shout, "There she comes!" And that is what we call dying.

(Source Unknown)

Contents

Acknowledgements

I first wish to thank my long time writing teachers, Nancy Beckett and Mel Levatino for always believing in my work and encouraging me to go forward despite my uncertainties and fears. They are the best. I also thank Terri Mathes for her kind and invaluable comments while editing my manuscript. My deepest thanks go to Dr. Nancy Angoff who kept Christine alive with her caring devotion and expertise. Special thanks go out to my husband Michael and children, Jason and Mika who always gave me the space and love I needed to complete this work. My heartfelt thanks to all my dear friends who have loved me unconditionally and have, over the years, supported whatever my heart desired. There can be no greater gift in friendship. Finally, I am truly grateful to have had Christine in my life for as long as I did, she has become my guiding light.

Introduction

For many reasons I resisted reading Connie Kiosse's book about her sister Christine who was my patient for six years. For so many reasons that I still do not fully understand I could not start. Connie says in the book that we originally agreed to write a story of three women coming to know themselves and each other in spite of the fact that Christine saw herself as a little girl lost. Christine forced me to examine myself as a woman about her same age, as someone who could have been on the examining table instead of standing next to it. And Connie, the writer, confronted me with the narrative, the story of my patient Christine, who ultimately died, and therefore, of myself, the physician who could not save her.

I came to medicine late in life, starting medical school at just under the age of forty, about the same time that Christine started to make her own decisions. So at an age when some physicians would be jaded, secure, understanding of their role, I met Christine and in her saw the vulnerability of myself. She was dying of AIDS already when I took over her care, and her timing – as it had been her whole life – was so badly off. She was too late to have avoided our early mistakes in sequential monotherapies and too early for the magic cocktails of multiple powerful medications that have truly saved and prolonged lives.

But Christine allowed me to do what I had already known I needed to do as a physician – help her die. "Do I have to be dying to find myself?" she asked. I have found myself as a physician who can help people die – because die we do in spite of the many, many ways in which we have learned and are learning to prolong life. But we die. When, how, under which circumstances, of course, we do not know.

Physicians are poor at prognosticating accurately. The night I visited Christine's home to have a conversation with her and some of her family about her wishes regarding care at the end of her life, I believed her death was months away. That night was over a year before she died. But that night she seemed at peace and ironically more alive and talkative than I had ever known her to be. At one point she disappeared into her bedroom to return with a box of old photographs that she shared with me. There were pictures of her as a beautiful fifteen- year old bride, eyes full of possibilities of life ahead of her. I saw her in ways I could never have imagined in her clinic visits. Glimpses of the person who was Christine included the sandy pinks and blues, the beach colors with which she decorated her home, her white fluffy cat, her ever present candles and her beloved grandson Mikey. These were gifts to a doctor wanting to respond to her needs in a way that suited her.

There are essential things about our patients that we wish we knew. There are also barriers to that knowledge – strange barriers that have nothing to do with the desire to know. Connie writes that Christine was "stuffing tears and dreams in a dark spot in the pit of her stomach." Her illness manifested itself in nausea, vomiting, abdominal pain and diarrhea. No wonder.

You think you know your patients. You want to believe you can know them from monthly or even weekly half hour clinic visits. You think you know yourself. "Do I have to be dying to find myself?" Christine asked. Through writing about her sister, Connie comes to know herself better. Through caring for the dying Christine, I came to know myself better – as a physician, as a person. I finally read *The Best of Friends*, at the beach. I am sure that Christine was there.

Nancy Angoff, M.D.
Associate Dean for Student Affairs,
Yale University School of Medicine,
Assistant Professor of Internal Medicine

Prologue

I knew no good would come from this early marriage. How could my father have thought this was a good idea? Why didn't I try and stop this ridiculous turn of events? I was always known as "the big one," or *e megale*, in Greek; I was supposed to make sure my siblings didn't get into trouble. How could my younger sister, Christine possibly have known how to be a good wife and mother? Did her premature dip into adulthood predict her premature death thirty-two years later? Or had her life accelerated at such a rate that it made more sense to think of it in cat years rather than human years?

That would've made Christine hundreds of years old. She called her last cat, Shag Meister T. Sassafras, her guardian angel. Shag watched her body age once the disease took over, watched her heart age with a wisdom beyond her years and he watched her soul soar with the freedom of wings, something he was forever chasing.

And so the story begins with my sister's life partly told by the two journals and notes she left behind. There's no denying she had a difficult life: an arranged marriage, three children by the age of twenty, divorce and single motherhood. There's no denying she wanted to leave life with a greater understanding of who she was. There's no denying she wanted to leave her girls with some of that understanding.

Of course our stories are entwined. I grew alongside my younger sister. The story must be about me too, how I slowly came to accept my spiritual self, a self long-neglected. How I came to see that death is not something to be feared.

Christine's wonderful doctor often said my sister grew because of her illness. She became the person she was meant to be, stronger, braver and more self-assured. I didn't understand. I didn't want to. I didn't like thinking that we got better at being human and then died. I'd often ask myself, Then what was the point? Why didn't we get more time so we could enjoy the life we'd created?

While writing about Christine's life I was also struggling with sudden deaths around me. How could a handsome younger cousin drop dead without warning? How could a beautiful Greek woman, my sister's age, die just a month before her oldest daughter's high school graduation? How could those left behind live without bitterness and regret?

Frequent travels to my Connecticut hometown continue, this time to visit my ailing mother, who's eighty-four and in a nursing home. Oh, how my heart tugs at her frailty, her reduced world, and her joy in seeing me. How will I manage this eventual death of my mother? How will I manage without the two women I grew up with?

Each time I visit Bridgeport I drive down State Street and stare at our old house. It bears no resemblance to the house it once was. Now it's painted yellow, the front door is broken, and the grass we weren't allowed to walk on no longer grows in the front yard. It's become a poor people's block. I stare and wonder how this house can be so alive in my imagination and so dead in reality. I wonder about the journey in between.

At the Beach

All I ever wanted was to be happy, with the simple things in life: a job/career that is rewarding, a loving warm family, good friends, a home that is truly Home Sweet Home. I see people like that around me and I ask myself, Do they know how lucky they are? How blessed they are? They seem to bicker about stupid things that really don't matter. Seems like they take most things for granted.

--Christine's Journal, 1997-8

The afternoon is gloriously warm and breezy. It's one of the last days of summer and I want my children to have a good time in the water. We've just arrived at our usual spot at Pratt Beach and I ask the skinny lifeguard why there aren't any people in the lake.

"No swimming today. Most of the lifeguards have gone back to college and there's not enough of us to cover the shifts, so sorry no swimming," he says.

"But you're here. Can't you watch the swimmers now?" I say, aware that the kid is not looking up from the wood and penknife he's got in his hands. He's carving something small. He's getting paid to carve?

"Sorry, that's what I was told, not to let anyone in the water right now. That's all I know. There's nothing I can do about it. Sorry."

I ignore his apology and look to the left and see two familiar older women. They're always here in their bikinis and orange skin. Don't they care about skin cancer? One of

1

the women must be in her seventies and the other one not too far behind. I suppose they could be sisters. They both have layers and layers of skin that fold over their large breasts and stomachs. The older one is wearing a pink and lime bikini and is lying down on a beach chair with green cups over her eyes and gold hoop earrings. She could be Bohemian or Slavic or Polish. The other woman is sitting on the sand next to her and all I see are huge breasts pushed high up towards her chin. She's wearing a turban and sunglasses. How can they flaunt their unbecoming flabby skin so freely? Aren't they embarrassed? Anyone who wears a bikini can't be that embarrassed. But then, isn't it wonderful that they aren't inhibited, that they don't care what others think about their flabby bodies?

In a few moments I look the other way and see several much younger women lying on towels with sunglasses and novels. They are wearing two-piece suits that fit. Decades ago I was one of these women, only farther south along the lakefront reading Doris Lessing's popular novel, *The Golden Notebook*. (Lonely women out for passion and self-fulfillment. I don't remember if they find either one in the 666 paperback pages.) These days I don't enjoy lying directly on the sand, I prefer to sit in a low chair and have my back supported. I also don't enjoy wearing any kind of suit; I prefer over the knee pants and a loose tank top.

"See, told you Mom," Mika says when I sit in my chair near her. "I told you we wouldn't be able to swim."

"Yes, you did sweetheart, but it's all right. Look we've practically got the beach to ourselves. We'll stay a couple of hours and then go." She turns back to her hole and continues to dig. She's always been the quieter one, my eleven-year-old who watches and waits, not unlike her mom. My thirteen- year-old son Jason is louder and not content to dig holes.

"We've got to find another beach that lets us swim. We never know if the big waves or the bacteria will close it down. Let's go someplace else," he says.

"No, we're fine here. Besides this is where Christine is," I say clutching my red and yellow starred beach bag which holds two photographs wrapped in plastic.

"Christine is wherever she wants to be now, she can fly like the seagulls," Jason says. He picks up some sticks he's brought and runs to the water's edge dipping them in.

My head arches from side to side as I look up at the clear sky. I feel enclosed in blue glass, my own hothouse dome. The horizon meets the water as the water moves gently back and forth, back and forth. It's like a sparkling emerald as small waves hit against the shore touching the smooth grains of clean sand stretching for miles in either direction. To the south I can see the Pier where a part of my sister's ashes were scattered five months after her death. Just beyond, the city skyline is visible, tall apartment buildings with the John Hancock on Michigan Avenue in clear view. To the north there's a busier beach with a playground and concession stand, and beyond are the large campuses of Loyola and Northwestern. I close my eyes and take a deep breath through my nose like I've learned to do in yoga. I take in the fishy, hot smells of the beach like those of a familiar lover. I hold them in for half a minute and then slowly exhale through my nose and remember my yoga teacher's mantra, "Keep your mouth closed! Your mouth is for eating not breathing." Sometimes I have a hard time keeping it closed.

I open my eyes and take another look around. The Bohemian sisters are talking in a language I cannot understand. The older one reaches for a spray bottle and starts to squirt water on her legs, arms and face. Her body glistens like a fish out of water. I reach into my bag and pull out the greasy sunscreen I hate putting on. I do it anyway and then call the kids and put some on them too. Then I pull out the photos. The large one is framed, the other is not. I place them on my lap side by side and stare into the images of my sister Christine and me.

We were happiest at the beach. Sand and water created an oasis where anything seemed possible. The first photograph was taken in the mid-sixties; it's black and white

3

with scalloped edges. My younger sister Christine and I were standing mid-thigh in Long Island Sound wearing silly looking bathing suits. I was fourteen in a tight, built-in bra kind of suit that must have belonged to my mother. Christine was ten in a sailor-type suit with a skirt and tie. I was so much taller than Christine. My left arm reached down behind her back and over her shoulder and her arm stretched up and barely reached my right shoulder. What was I thinking? Surely even then I was biding my time waiting to leave my East Coast home four years later. What was my sister thinking? Surely even then she must have been biding her time too; little did she know that she had less time to plan her escape.

There's a large space between us in the photograph; a small person could easily have fit under our stretched interlocked arms. Instead, the Sound flowed through on its way to the Atlantic. What else might have floated between us? My right arm was away from my body and my fingers were wide apart as if to splash away an unpleasant thought. Christine's left arm and hand rested firmly alongside her body as if to keep herself steady. We were together then. Waiting for our lives to begin.

Suddenly the Madonna chapel clock behind me gongs one, two, three times. Seagulls appear next to us, waiting to be fed. I don't have anything to give them. I worry one of them may be my sister's spirit and quickly give the kids five dollars to run over to the concession stand for snacks. The gulls wait patiently and I return to the time when I still had a sister.

The second photograph is framed and taken in 1995. We were standing at the edge of the Pacific Ocean, four thousand miles away from home. (By then I was forty-seven with a long-time husband and two small children. Christine was forty-three with an ex-husband and three grown girls.) The picture is nicely framed in ornate pewter and engraved. What strikes me now is how we've got the same pose in both photos. I was still the one on the left, Christine on the right. My right hand was still away from my body and I was still

4

reaching down to hold onto my sister. Her right hand was slightly raised this time and she didn't have to reach up as far to hold onto me. We were wearing sunglasses to cover our squinting eyes and large T-shirts to cover oversized bellies. We were much closer together and our arms link in the same way, only now it wasn't such a stretch. Behind us was a huge dark boulder that stopped the water around our feet from moving through smoothly.

What were we thinking only seven years ago? Of course I remember the moment. We wanted to stop and put our feet into the ocean – to smell the salt, to feel the chill, to be in something that would remain long after we were gone. Of course I remember the joy my sister felt in finally arriving at her Mecca. "Connie, I can't believe we're here; we're here in California and our feet are in the ocean. I want to stay forever."

I'm still here. Christine's not. She died a slow death three years ago back in our home state of Connecticut. A kind of death we never imagined for any of us, death caused by AIDS. Not unlike the plague that suddenly swallowed my mother's father months before she was born, the influenza epidemic of 1918. That epidemic took millions too, only it disappeared as quickly as it came. We grew up not believing our grandfather had died of something as simple as the flu. Now our children grow up believing there was never a time without AIDS.

Jason and Mika appear with hot dogs, a bag of chips and drinks.

"How come you brought those pictures to the beach?" Jason says. "They'll get all wet and sandy and then you'll have to throw them away."

Mika looks over and says, "Maybe Mom wanted Christine to be with us. She loved the beach too, you know."

I cover the photos with a towel and wonder how my children got to be so wise. We eat our hot dogs. I break off bits of the bun and throw them out for the seagulls. They rush to our side and start to fight over the pieces. Jason and

Mika throw out chips and soon we've got dozens of gulls surrounding us. Next time we'll bring a bag of old bread.

After we've eaten we each enter our own worlds again. I remove the towel and look into the framed photo and recall how Christine gave it to me for my fiftieth birthday a year before she died in 1999. She was very sick then, but she had her daughter in Las Vegas enlarge the photo and search for a suitable frame. The stylish cursive slants to the right and reads, *Sea Sisters Forever, Happy 50th, Love, Christine.* On my birthday she called and said, "I hope you like it. I'm not crazy about the picture, I've got that silly Tweety pie T-shirt and my hair is flat, but you look good. I couldn't find another and I wanted it to be of us in the ocean. Tina picked out the frame. I hope you like it."

"I love it. I think you look better than I do," I said. "And I love the pewter." I'm relieved to remember happier times by the Pacific.

California was where my young fun-loving grandfather had gotten sick with influenza. I think he owned a restaurant around Los Angeles and lived with my pregnant grandmother and their three children. (They had come from Greece not long before and from many accounts were wildly happy together.) My grandfather knew he was dying and asked to be brought to his parent's house in Massachusetts. The family traveled four thousand miles by train, and my grandfather died days later in his mother's house. My mother was born several months later. She never liked the beach, the sand or the water. She sat under a tree on the grass waiting for us to return, hungry, tired and wet.

I gaze at both photographs, the only ones we ever took in either ocean, and I'm amazed at the distance my sister and I have traveled, together and apart. In the end I'd like to believe we were more together than apart. Certainly I became a better sister and a better person while we slowly navigated the unknown waters of Christine's illness. That journey took eight years; from the time she was diagnosed with the virus in 1991 to the time of her death on Father's Day in 1999.

My arms tingle with the memory of her last breath. I bounce up from my chair and start walking towards the pier. I turn my head back and say, "I need to stretch my legs, watch our stuff." I don't wait for a reply as I pick up my pace and watch my feet sink in and out of the water. Within minutes I'm on the pier and halfway to the end. I stop at the slight indentation in the cable railing; I hold onto it with both hands and stare out at the lake. Could any ash particle still be floating nearby? Almost three years later, could an ash have clung to the wooden beams holding up this pier?

I tighten my grip on the railing and close my eyes. Christine, are you here? Christine, are you floating around me? Christine, remember the cold windy morning we dropped you off here?

My head whirls and suddenly I feel a tap on my shoulder.

"Hey lady, are you all right?"

I open my eyes and look at the young girl next to me. She's wearing a large sun hat and a polka dot swimsuit. I don't know what to say, so I don't say anything.

"Hey, you are all right aren't you? I can call my dad up ahead and he can help you get to a doctor."

"I don't need a doctor. I was only closing my eyes and remembering," I say, pleased at the concern of this young stranger.

"Well, I like to do that too; I like to remember all the good stuff," she says.

"Sometimes it's not only the good stuff that comes up, sometimes it's the sad stuff," I say as I look down at her large eyes and red cheeks.

"I don't like feeling sad, so I don't close my eyes for that," she says, then runs to catch up to her father.

I watch her and think maybe she's right. Maybe keeping my eyes open is a better way to see Christine. Just then I'm reminded of a favorite poem (attributed by some to a Native American prayer) she had re-worded, so like Christine to change it to make it hers. A poem she gave me months before she died.

Do not think of me and cry
I am not dead; I did not die.
I am the gentle summer breeze that blows
I am one of many stars that glow
I am warm sunlight shining on your face
I am the sound of gentle waves on the beach –
My favorite place.
I did not leave – I am still here.
Think of me and I will be there.
Don't think of me and cry
I am not dead. I did not die.

The words linger gently around my heart. I walk off the pier and slowly head towards my children.

When I return Jason asks me, "Mom, how can you like the water but not even own a bathing suit? How come you never swim?"

At first I'm surprised, as I usually am by his candor. It sounds silly to me too. "I love to watch the water and it's very relaxing for me to be around it. I guess I don't really like to get my body all wet and I'm not a good swimmer."

"Christine can go wherever she wants now; she's the boss now, isn't she?" Mika asks.

"Yes, she's the boss. Her soul travels to all her favorite places," I say, suddenly aware of my longing to return to either coast, to return to the wild salt waters so unlike the tame clear lake.

Somehow I wound up in the Midwest. Often my spirit travels to the coastlines: to the eastern coastline where I grew up, where my sister lived and died, where my mother and brothers remain; to the western coastline, where longtime friends live, where I feel at home. Sometimes I wonder if I'd settled in mid-country to learn about balance, to learn how to live with the unpredictability of life and death.

Often I visualize the shape of America, its rough edges and the vastness of the land within its borders. I watch with curiosity from a high place and wonder how life will play itself out: will I live a long life? Will I die a sudden death? Will it matter so terribly much in the end?

In the end my sister's life and death was a precursor to mine. In the end my sister's death has become the defining death, the one by which I measure all deaths before and after hers. I ache to know how well others hold up to her brave and peaceful end. I read the obituaries and wonder: did the person feel fulfilled? Did the person say good-bye? Did the person die peacefully? Of course I have no way of knowing, but often times I worry about the dying. I imagine a chorus of desires unsung. I imagine a life gone – poof – just like the bird in a magician's hat. It's usually a dove, isn't it, white lovely and amazing.

Life itself is amazing. So much has changed but so much has remained the same. We're in a new century, one that my sister missed by six months. We're in deeper world trouble and AIDS has taken millions of lives around the globe. The oceans will outlive this century, the troubles and the diseases of the world. The oceans my sister and I once stood in will be around for eons. Maybe someday I'll even learn to swim in them.

Promises

Ignorance breeds fear. That's why I'm trying to explain things, to relieve some of the fears people may have. Who was I? What was my hard life about? But I must write it down. How else will they know when I'm not here anymore?

I was a lousy big sister. I didn't want to take my little sister Christine with me anywhere. I didn't want any reminders of home. For as long as I can remember I avoided being around her. Later - much later - at the end of her life I made up for it. I became her companion in death. It's not something I took to easily. It's not something I ever dreamed I'd do. It's not something I will ever regret.

In the last weeks of her life during the spring of 1999 I remember wheeling her outside to the beautiful gardens of her Hospice home in Connecticut. It was a warm day and I parked the chair in a sunny patch of blue sky. I pulled up a chair and placed it next to her. Christine was quiet. She didn't have a lot to say. But then she had never been the talkative one. It was up to me to bring up the important and not so important stuff. I went for the unimportant first.

"What else can I bring from your apartment? Any CD's you want to hear? Any photo albums?" I remembered her new love of country western singers like Reba McIntyre and hoped they'd offer solace in her dying days.

"You've gone to so much trouble already. Just sit here with me."

"Well I'll bring something – I can't not come without anything. How about some jelly donuts and coffee from Dunkin Donuts?"

"If you want."

"Okay, I'll bring that by in the morning." Connecticut was the only place where I could get white powdered jelly donuts; they didn't have those in Chicago. Just like they didn't have maple walnut ice cream or sauerkraut on hot dogs. It had been thirty-three years since I'd left my hometown of Bridgeport, Connecticut, and the world no longer felt like it would go on forever. I went for what I wanted to know. "Remember I said someday I'd write a book about you? Remember I said Dr. Angoff thought it was a great idea and she might write something too? Do you have any thoughts on what you'd like it to be called?"

"I can't imagine it. Who would want to read about me?"

"Lots of people would. I love stories about real people. Not the famous ones; they'll be remembered anyway. Why do they want to take over writing too? Try and think on a title for the book." We sat in silence for the next ten minutes. I looked over at Christine's closed face and wondered where her heart was now. Maybe it was with her spirit slowly seeping out of her ravaged body, a body weighing no more than 80 pounds, a body unable to stand on its own.

"Maybe it should be called *Little Girl Lost*," she said in a whisper, her eyes still closed, facing the sun.

"Do you feel lost now?" I said trying to sound normal while my heart took extra beats and my left breast moved up and down as if it had a pulse of its own.

"I was lost before I even started out. I see myself on the beach wandering forever. Wandering like a seagull, not taking up much space at all. Only without the wings."

"I don't know. You've done a lot. You raised three girls mostly on your own, you've traveled like you wanted to and you've lived by the beach. Dr. Angoff thinks you've done wonderfully all these years. She says you've become your own person, doing what you want and not what others want you to do. She's very proud of you. And so am I."

"I'm almost dead. I did what I had to do. If I could do my life over I'd do it differently and leave right away like you did. You were always the smart one."

"I got the chance and you didn't. I don't know why that was. Maybe it should be sub-titled, *Big Girl Found*," I said hoping to get a smile out of her, hoping she wouldn't be mad at me, her older sister, for living longer. I smiled but she didn't.

"Do I have to be dying to find myself?" Christine's eyes opened and stared into mine. Her eyes were now her biggest feature. "I don't know. I just don't think dying is something to be admired for."

I looked over at Christine about to ask her something else but she'd fallen asleep. Her face was slumped onto her shoulders and her mouth was open. I reached over with my balled up sweater to make a pillow under her cheek. I didn't want her to wake up with a cramp in her neck. I didn't want her to wake up and regret she was still alive.

I hadn't brought anything to read, so I looked around as my heart spoke to my head. Sometimes there was so much to talk about, but at other times there was nothing left to say. Death was all around and the silence was filled with unanswered questions. How did it feel to be dying? How much longer would my sister have? How would she die? An older woman's hospital bed was being wheeled out and put under a large tree nearby. She had several blankets on her despite the warm temperatures. I stared at her small face crowned with stray strands of white hair. Someone lighted a cigarette and handed it to her. The old woman took it, put it in her mouth and sucked on it for a while before letting out the smoke. I was surprised they allowed smoking there. Another skinny younger man wheeled himself out and passed us. I nodded and he nodded back without a smile. Some healthy looking people came out and sat nearby but they weren't talking. They must have been visitors, like me. I waited for my sister to awaken, thankful that on this day she would.

On this same visit I asked her again about her wishes to be cremated. I wanted to make sure she hadn't changed her mind. I wanted to make sure I was doing the right thing. My mother, brothers and the Greek priest were against it. (When I mentioned this wish to my mother she had the priest call to try and persuade not to agree with my sister's decision. When I asked him if it was a sin to be cremated, at first he hesitated but then said no it wasn't but it was a tradition to be buried.) I didn't think her daughters were crazy about the idea either. The middle one Tina asked, "Where will I go to see my mother? Where will I go to sit and talk with her?" When I had mentioned this to Christine she said, "Tell her to go to the ocean; that's where I'll be. I don't want people looking down at me. I don't want people looking down at the dirt, that's not where I'll be."

When I asked this time she simply said, "Yes, yes, I still want to be burned and scattered. I don't want to rot in the earth – I'd feel too trapped down there. I want to be free."

For most of my adult years I had confused religion with spirituality. I had dismissed the church and its religion as irrelevant. Too dated, too old, too rigid. What I hadn't known before my sister's diagnosis of AIDS was that our spirits and souls are separate and free entities. Separate and free from organized religion. What my sister's dying years gave me was part of my soul, part of my spirit, back. Of course there was no way to have known that ten years ago when I first heard of her HIV infection. I hadn't known what the path ahead might look like. I only heard her fear and my resistance, her fear for her life and my resistance to going down that road of death. The call came in February of 1991.

She said, "I've got something to tell you, but I don't know how to say it."

"What's wrong?" I said as I reached for the rocking chair behind me and sat down. I re-positioned the phone to my left ear and waited. What was wrong now: One of the girls in trouble? She'd lost her job and had no money? Was her old boyfriend still giving her problems? Nothing had ever come easy to my sister, nothing except trouble. There was a moment of silence and I looked around the dining room and noticed the bright yellow flowers on the table nearby. I stared at their brilliance and wished my sister's life was less chaotic.

"It's Sal, I got a call from his brother. Remember how I told you he was acting nuts and I had to leave? Remember how scared the girls and I got? I didn't know what was the matter with him."

"What did his brother have to say?" Images of curly headed Sal appeared. I smiled and then caught myself; I was still pissed at him for scaring my sister. Before the image faded I saw him hanging on Christine with a happy grin on his face. They had been so in love. They had thought it was a forever kind of love.

"He called last week and told me to go get a blood test right away."

"A blood test, for what Christ's sake? What's the matter with him? Does he have gonorrhea?" I curled the phone cord around my fingers, walked into the kitchen and stared out the window at the dark red brick wall next door.

"I wish. It's worse than that. It's a lot worse. I can't even believe it. Except that his brother doesn't usually joke around. He says Sal has AIDS."

"How could he get that?" I uncurled the cord and drummed my fingers against the counter top. This was going to be a lot worse than I had thought. This was big time trouble.

"I don't know, but his brother says I should get myself tested. I'm sure I'm all right, but I had the test done yesterday and I have to go back next week for the results."

"Where did you go? Who did you go with?" I said needing to fill the space with questions so I wouldn't have to feel the terror creeping up my backside.

14

"I went to the women's health clinic nearby and I went by myself. I haven't told anyone yet. Not even the girls."

"How the hell did he get AIDS? How the hell could he have gotten himself in this mess?" In 1991 I didn't know anyone with the virus or AIDS. It was ten years into the epidemic but I, like most people, didn't even know the difference between the virus and AIDS. Then it was still largely considered a gay man's disease, a disease I couldn't imagine living with although I'd been scared for my gay friends. I had thought the call might someday come from one of them, but never ever from my traditional, working class, straight, non-smoking, non-drinking little sister.

"I don't know how he got it. I caught him with a needle once but he promised me he'd never ever do it again. I believed him. I believed he'd change for me and for us. But I'm all right. I'm sure I'm safe. It doesn't get women like me as much as it does gay guys."

"You're probably right. But I'll call you next Sunday to hear about the results unless you call me before that. Call me anytime." I said trying to sound like we were talking about a regular blood test.

February 17th was the next Sunday. Now, a decade later I search the bookcases near my computer to find the engagement calendar for that year. After a few minutes I see it along with the others I've saved. Nineteen ninety-one's calendar title is "The Subject is Women." I flip through the days filled with holidays, birthdays, dinners, friends, outings with my almost two-year-old son Jason, and book group's *Animal Dreams* by Barbara Kingsolver. I'd just finished reading that book about two sisters and adored it. The story made me think about my own sister and how much closer we'd gotten over the years. I remember feeling disbelief while reading: I hadn't anticipated the death of the younger sister. It seemed to come out of the blue.

I continue flipping through the weeks and am pleased that I've saved my appointment books. I can easily pinpoint dates and events. For the week of February 11th there's a 16th

15

century painting by an Italian called "Venus and Cupid." A plump naked woman is reclining on pillows with an erect left breast nipple. Her stomach protrudes and her belly button is a deep cavern. She's holding a chubby baby boy who's staring into her eyes. He's naked, too, and his tiny penis is visible although I have to look twice to make sure that's what it was and not a speck of dirt or a marker dot. It's mournfully erotic.

There was nothing erotic about the conversation my sister and I had about her blood test results. There was plenty to be mournful about. Chilling waves went through my skull as my sister told me, *"Yes, I have the HIV virus."* I don't recall what else we said. I only recall thinking everyone who gets AIDS dies within a short period of time. I was ready to scream. *NO, NO not my little sister, NO!* Instead I hung up after I promised to call her in a couple of days once she had made an appointment with the clinic.

What my heart screamed after the call was, No, no, no! I don't want to know anything about AIDS. No, no, no! Why weren't you more careful? How could you have been so dumb? How could you have let this curly headed jerk fuck you up?

I didn't talk with anyone that day, not even my husband Michael. I didn't want to make the terrible news more real by saying it out loud. I didn't want to be part of the millions affected by this plague. It took me a while before I was able to tell my friends and even longer to tell my family. I don't remember how long. I only remember the hurt and embarrassment that this disease should infect my sister. She hadn't done anything bad. My head and heart quickly filled with questions. Why her and not someone who lived more dangerously? Why not someone who acted like they didn't care whether they lived or died, like a drug addict or a prostitute or some jerk who'd slept with hundreds of guys? How could my hard-luck sister have such a dreaded disease?

Two weeks later I flew out to Connecticut to go to the clinic with my sister. My mother and nieces wondered why I'd come out in such a hurry. Christine didn't want

16

anyone else to know, not even her fairly new sweetheart of a boyfriend, Andy. I felt excited but burdened by her decision; excited that she trusted me, but burdened by the responsibility. *How would I ever get through this terrible time with her?* How will we manage to live normal lives knowing what we knew?

Flipping through the calendar pages of 1991, I noted so much life and so much death. Our daughter Mika was born. I joined Concerned and United Parents to search for my first daughter, long lost to adoption. A dear older friend Taka died of cancer. A longtime friend and former partner of my younger brother, Dixie died in a freak car accident. It was sudden and shocking. I used the bad news to reassure Christine she wasn't the only one with death lurking about. (It was something I'd do often in the coming years, from Gilda Radner's to Michael Landon's to Princess Diana's premature deaths. "See, see, see? Anybody can die at any moment; no one is safe. I was not aware that I was excluding myself from the "anybody" list.)

At the end of 1991 Christine turned forty and I invited her to come visit. I picked her up at O'Hare airport and surprised her by taking her to the fancy Fairmont Hotel in downtown Chicago where Michael and I had celebrated my fortieth three and a half years earlier. We drank champagne, ate linguine with clam sauce and pretended we were on top of the world.

"Connie, this place is so beautiful. If only we could stay here and not ever have to leave. We could order room service and watch old movies and sleep all we wanted. I could even live in the bathroom it's so big!" Christine said even though her stomach was cramped and she was lying on her side with her feet propped up to her chest. Severe stomach problems plagued her for the rest of her life.

"Don't you want to meet Mika? You're going to love her; she's like a kewpie doll, so chubby and adorable. And Jason and Michael are waiting for you too." Then, my long-awaited daughter was only seven months and Jason two and a half. Life at home was exhausting, especially the day after

Christmas and I'd left Michael with the mess once again. I remember I was anxious to get home.

"I want to see Mika, but I don't want to leave here either! Let's just stay until the last possible moment. Hey let me call Andy and let him try to guess where I am. He'll never believe it!"

"Sure, go ahead and call."

Christine picked up the phone and went to the window to stare out at Lake Michigan. She dialed and I watched as she shouted,

"Hey guess where I'm calling from? You'll never guess in a million years!" She let Andy guess several times before she told him where she was – high up in the clouds without a care in the world. It did my heart good to see her so excited about living and forgetting about the nearness of death.

Now, ten years later I no longer exclude myself from that possibility of near death. I could go in a heartbeat. Sometimes in bed my spirit travels outside my body and into the infinite space beyond my window. My head spins and I make myself sick with the thought I will someday simply cease to exist. The trees outside my window will live, the house will live, people around me will live. I'm sick in a terrifying kind of way. When I was a child I remember dizzying thoughts of nonexistence. Only then I soothed myself with, "Don't think about that now, you've got years and years before you have to worry about disappearing." I'd rock my mind and body back to sleep with promises of all the tomorrows ahead of me.

Now more of my life is behind me than in front of me. The spinning should terrify me more, but it no longer does. Watching death up close with Christine has eased the terror within me. Watching death up close has brought something greater than myself into being, something I never considered before: the possibility of something greater, an afterlife, a forever existence.

These possibilities didn't come easily. I fought them with logic and common sense. I fought them with the resistance of my younger self. I fought them with all my heart and soul, until I had no choice, until I could no longer merely watch death; until I thought my heart would break from the unfairness of my sister's fate.

I began the first chapter of my memoir, *It's All Greek to Me*, with my sister's death day and ended the book with her birthday that same year, 1999. She surrounds my life chapter after chapter as I travel back and forth in time. Now I surround hers in similar circles. Who was my sister? Who was/am I in relation to her? Who am I in relation to myself without her?

And what do I see now in 2001, when I begin this book that I didn't see earlier? Maybe our growing up years weren't that dissimilar after all. She was just as miserable as I was. She may have had it worse as a middle child with no one paying much attention. I as the oldest got lots of attention. Her life was filled with grief – the same grief I thought I had escaped. Her life became finite and I've come to see, so has mine.

The gift of her death. I cannot write "gift" without a stab of guilt. How could her death be a gift? Certainly in the end it was when her body was so wasted. The gift may be in the journey I took with her to the death we must all face. The gift may be in the presence of self I felt whenever I was with her. The gift may be in my becoming a spiritual being once again. Books say children are naturally spiritual but are quickly trained to distrust their hearts. I suppose I must have connected to many worlds as a child – I must have imagined all sorts of wonderful adventures before I started school. It's not something I remember. I also suppose many of us spend our lives trying to regain that innocence of spirit.

Staying fully alive became my sister's main mission during the last nine years of her life. Christine's death story must also tell her life story. For how could someone die without being alive first?

Over the years I'd sent countless fancy journals with the plea, "Write something down. It might make you feel better, it might be a release for you," all the while being aware of my own craving to have her writings after she was gone. I cradle her black and red dotted journal like I cradled my first baby before letting her go. The journal is 8 ½ by 5 ½ inches long with a long –haired black and white cat on the cover not unlike her old cat Shag. I let go of the keyboard and use my arms to squeeze the book closer to my heart as if the words could mesh with mine and become one story. I pull the journal away from my heart and stare into the eyes of the old cat lying on a white and black tiled floor. If he could speak he might say, *"I'm all you've got now. Tread wisely."*

I open the book and the leaf page holds the date: August 1997. The night she thought she would die. I turn another page and she begins her story.

My first memory of anything was when I was in kindergarten. My teacher's name was Miss Skelly. She had bright candy apple red long fingernails and lips to match. Her black hair was pulled back tightly to a neat ponytail. She was nice and I recall having fun in her class. I became good friends with Margie Marko – she lived a few houses away from mine growing up. I remember crying when we had to separate because we were going to first grade. She went in one classroom and I went to another.

I also remember all of a sudden being called Dorothy. I hated that name, my father thought it up. Kids in school teased me and called me "Dorothy from Kansas" or "Where's Toto?" I had no idea what they were talking about. I never saw "The Wizard of Oz" until I watched it with my daughters while they were growing up.

I never did much fun stuff growing up – seems like we weren't allowed to laugh and have fun – too much yelling and screaming going on – mostly my father. I hated it when he was home. The one place we did have fun was at the beach. To this day I love it.

Going over to Margie's house was fun - she had the best toys! She had a Barbie doll with all the clothes and case to go with it and a beautiful Barbie house. I loved playing there. Margie would ask her mom for a dime and "one for Dorothy too" and we would go down to "John's" the neighborhood store and buy Popsicle's and potato chips. I loved when we would watch scary movies on Saturday afternoons and make popcorn. We became the best of friends.

Christine didn't die that night. She had almost another two years of life left. But she wrote through that August night like she never had before. Thirty-three pages. I remember her showing me these pages soon after she wrote them. I was scared and I was excited. Scared that this might be her last testament and excited that she was finally writing in something besides the small, gray journal that kept track of her drug treatments. I didn't know she also had written in a yellow legal sized pad until after her death when I found it among her papers. I took the two journals and the note pad and packed them into my suitcase. It's what I treasure most now that she's gone.

The summer after Christine died I sent Margie a copy of the obituary I had printed and put on large cards with an ornate rose border. I remember bringing my children to Kinko's while I chose the design and then waited for the copying to be done. Nothing looked right, not the smiling kid behind the counter; not the traditional stationary and not the way I was leaning against the back wall. Jason and Mika stood close enough to catch me if I fell too much to one side.

"Mom, how come you're crying in the store? Is it cause we've been waiting too long?" Jason asks.

"Leave her alone, don't you know she's tired?" Mika says.

"It's all right, don't worry. I'm thinking about Christine and how I can't believe we won't see her again this summer like we usually do," I say. Suddenly I remember

21

something Jason said long ago, "Mom, can we make a special machine so all of us in the world will not die?" I smiled and said, "Well no, sweetheart, what would happen to the others waiting to be born – where would they go?" After a long silence he said, "I don't know, I guess we have to make room."

I suppose remembering is a way of making room in our hearts. I so wanted everyone to know what a brave woman my sister had been. I wanted her first best girlfriend to know that she was not forgotten. Margie wrote back quickly.

I am sad to hear of Christine's death. I often thought of her whenever I went back into my memories of childhood. Dorothy (oops) forgive me for that is how I knew her, knowing even when we were younger she used to tell me she didn't like her name. I truly felt a loss in my heart when Maria told me. I have such good memories of her and I can laugh and smile at all of them. She was my first best friend and it was so sad when she got married and moved away. I never heard from her again. And then we saw each other a few years ago at a wake and I gave her my phone number but we never got together. I wish we had! I remember she and I would go down in your cellar and talk about when we got a car and were sixteen we were going to travel all over the country and for money we would find a nice town, work washing dishes, Ha!Ha!, and be waitresses, then when we had enough money we would drive on and do it all over again. And we said we would never get married but have boyfriends and find a rich one and move down south. What dreams we had.

I remember our dark cellar was the only place we could have some privacy. There were no closed doors allowed in our two-bedroom wood framed house. The second floor was rented out to boarders by the week and then eventually to a family with two women and two boys. The dimly lit cellar was divided into three areas. The front space had clotheslines,(we never had a dryer) the second smaller room had two huge barrels where my Dad made his red wine in the fall, and the third area had secret dark corners where unknown things were stored with tall piles of old newspapers stacked everywhere. My parents didn't want us down there, but we crept down the stairs anyway whispering secrets.

The phrase, *We became the best of friends,* keeps repeating in my heart, the best of friends, the best of friends. Don't the best of friends help one another out of impossible situations, soothe aching hearts, don't they eventually become family? Would the best of friends have taken that road trip on their own? I imagine Christine and Margie would've gone and had the kind of adventures we watched cute George Maharis (a Greek!) and the not as cute Martin Milner have every week on the popular Route 66 series in the early '60's. The open road was so romantic and full of possibilities. The girls would've found a way to make their road trip come true. In the series the end scene always finished with the two guys waving goodbye to their new-found friends, smiling and getting into their convertible. Now I imagine a similar kind of journey, only this time it'd be the girls breaking hearts in those small towns on their way out west in their Stingray Corvette.

Child Bride and Mother

My mother went right along with whatever my father said; she didn't stand up for me! She knew I wasn't happy, but I guess that wasn't important to her. I remember being really angry at her for that. How could you give away your daughter to a total stranger you don't even know? He was Greek, that's how.

Christine and I became friends after I got married at thirty-one and ached for children of my own. I began paying attention to my cute nieces and their mother, attention I hadn't given any of them in my twenties, especially after my father arranged a marriage for her when she was fifteen. Mostly I'd given that attention to myself, and my struggle to find a home of my own. During the 1980's we'd talk on the phone for hours and slowly our adult relationship evolved. My marriage was beginning and Christine's was ending. I couldn't wait to be an at-home mom and my sister couldn't wait to leave home and go out into the work world. I envied my sister's daughters; they were beautiful. My heart ached to know how my birth daughter Alethea was growing up. The daughter I'd given to adoption at birth, only months after my first niece was born in 1969. Was she happy, was she healthy and was she nearby? (Years later I found the answer was yes to all three questions.)

Visits back and forth became commonplace as my nieces grew older and we'd send them plane tickets to come visit us during summer vacations. Michael and I took them around the city to The Art Institute, the Shedd Aquarium and Chicago Fest at Navy Pier. I imagined doing the same with our children, children we weren't to have until ten years after our wedding. Children I couldn't imagine having when I was younger like my sister.

Christine and I would often talk about our lousy childhoods, how terrible and lonely, how unloved and unappreciated we felt.

I don't like to harp on the bad, sad parts of growing up, but the physical and verbal abuse by my father was traumatizing to me – it still bothers me to this day – but I try to leave the past behind and tell myself he did the best he could.

My parents came over from Europe; my mother from Greece, my father from up north, Macedonia. They didn't speak English very well, but I think my father did very well for himself – owning his own business and his own home, plus renting out apartments in the house he owned next door to ours.

I don't think my father was happy with the way his life turned out. Maybe that's why he was always so miserable.

I remember a time when we were all gathered around the kitchen table. We were all under twelve years old. Mom was at the sink piling up dirty dishes and had her back to us. After dinner Pop liked to test us on how smart we were.

"What did you learn in school today?" he said with a grin. My mom stopped clanking the dishes. The four of us stopped fidgeting. I prayed he wouldn't pick me.

"Nobody talks when they're supposed to talk," he said to my mother's back.

"Christine, where is Australia and what kind of weather is there now?"

I looked over at my sister whose head was bowed down. She mumbled, "I don't know, some place far away."

"How come? How come you don't know anything? You don't listen to the teacher that's why." He stood up, lifted his right hand with the ring on it and Whack! Red streaks appeared on Christine's left cheek and then Whack! on her other cheek. She put her hands up to her face and held them there. My brothers were stones and my mom didn't turn from the sink. I was mad at her for that.

He looked at us, still standing, with eyes wide open and said, *Kapu de katz!* or "shit-head" in Vlachi, and held his breath for a moment. Suddenly spit flew in Christine's direction. It landed on her bare arm, a wet glob of hatred. No one moved. He turned and walked out the back door. I handed Christine a used napkin, but by then the glob had run down her arm and onto the tablecloth. There was nothing visible to wipe up.

I suppose this anger is the blood price many immigrant families pay when they replant their lives on the other side of the world. I remember during my twenties I'd brag about my lousy childhood. "Hey if I had it good, I wouldn't have had to leave home. I wouldn't be wandering around searching for answers. I would be a good shoe-maker's daughter living by my parents, and giving them lots of grandchildren." I remember feeling righteous about this statement: *Hey, I'm a tough girl ready to fight. Don't mess with me.*

Except at school. No one messed with me there. I adored school, teachers and books. School was another life, a life filled with warm rooms, friendly people and pages of soothing words. Unlike home, engulfed with the fires of anger and disappointment, where we had no books to cradle our lonely hearts. I was the big one who did well in school. I led and my brothers and sister were to follow. Teachers like Miss Kantor expected the same love from them and they would often hear, "Why can't you be more like your big sister?" Of course I loved it, being considered the smart one. The one who'd go far out into the world. If that meant leaving them behind well, it wasn't my fault was it? There's no way around it: I was a smug pain in the ass.

I remember not liking school. I was never really good at anything besides spelling. I went every day and got perfect attendance awards for about three years. (I think that was because I didn't want to stay home.) I hated being home and always remember wanting to leave – My sister Connie felt that way too – She was 3½ years older than me and when she graduated high school she left.

Connie and I never had our own room. We slept on Castro convertibles in the dining room – it was awful – no privacy at all. Sometimes at night when it was real late and dark, we would talk – seemed like for hours and that felt good.

Until I read these lines I had no recollection of those nights. Suddenly an image appears. I'm lying in bed with the covers up to my chin. My head is turned away from my sister. She's whispering to me and I answer with short words, only wanting to sleep. Did we talk about school, teachers, clothes, and boys? I remember the excitement in her voice, but I don't remember a single word.

I do remember more words my father would fling at us in anger. Ugly words in Greek or Vlachi: a spoken language with no written words – languages he shared with my mother but not with us. Foreign words like: *glara* and *touvla,* translating roughly to: "crazy woman and brick headed." Words meant to wound us into submission. Words meant to unleash the anger and disappointment our father felt at having to work as a shoemaker. He left Macedonia to get away from his cobbler career. Later we learn he dreamed of becoming an accountant and that he loved to work with numbers.

My mother and father were always hard working – my mother, at home caring for my sister and me and my two brothers – she would also paint and clean the apartments that my father rented out. My father worked at his shoe store, repairing shoes six days a week. On hot summer nights and Sundays he would tend to his tomato plants, it seemed like there were hundreds of them! I loved the smells that came from the garden and to this day whenever I smell that sweet aroma of tomatoes, it reminds me of that garden.

I left Christine and home while she was still in high school. Terrible things began to happen. Would I have been able to stop some of them? Would I have been able to protect my sister? My head tells me no, no, no I couldn't have helped myself, let alone someone else. Every now and then my heart says yes, yes, yes, I could have prevented fate from taking its course, even if it meant butting heads with my father, the architect of her misery.

My high school days weren't any better – couldn't go anywhere or do anything. So I did what I was taught early in life- sneak out. I was about fourteen and started liking this boy Dominic. He wasn't handsome – he had terrible acne- but he had the most beautiful eyes I ever saw. I would go over to his house after school and we would talk, go to the park, and wow, the affection I was starving for!

My father found out after awhile. Boy, was he furious!

I guess about this time he thought he would marry me off – I didn't want to get married – I was only fifteen! I wanted to finish high school, I told him that and also I didn't love this person he had chosen for me. He told me that I would in time. I resisted. He probably was afraid I would get pregnant or leave home like my sister did.

For the first time I was allowed to go out with "Theo" – he was a Greek merchant marine who had jumped ship and wanted to stay in this country, so he had a stake in the deal too. My father promised to pay all his immigration fees etc. He helped him out tremendously financially. He bought him a brand new car (although I think it was part of the bribe for me.) I was never really impressed with jewelry, but Theo bought me an expensive diamond engagement ring.

After many weeks of resisting, I finally gave in. Well, I thought, this was my ticket out! I made Theo promise me

that if we got married, we would leave Connecticut for good.
He agreed.

Did my leaving make it harder on my sister, my
brothers and my mother? Did my leaving create an empty
space where heartache had more room to grow? I was the
one to leave and I was also the one to get pregnant. My
parents' worst fear had come true: a daughter pregnant and
unmarried. I suppose women have been stoned to death for
less. Luckily I was a thousand miles away and didn't have to
live with their despair. I had enough of my own to keep me
occupied.

Theo was lots of fun, he loved to laugh, tell jokes, be
the center of attention. I never knew that kind of life. We
would go out to Greek nightclubs, but I was really shy and
didn't like dancing. Theo would get up all by himself on the
dance floor – what a show he would put on! Theo worked in
restaurants and he made lots of money and he loved to throw
it around – wow – I never knew that either, my father being
really tight with his money.
I really had no idea how to live a healthy, happy life
and relationship – what did I know at fifteen! Theo was
really affectionate too. I loved that, he would always kiss and
hug me and tell me he loved me. Well, I figured, he was a
decent person. He loved his family back in Greece, he would
often call his mother, brothers and sister, and they were very
nice fun- loving people also.
My mother loved the fact he was Greek. She loved his
joking ways, money spending, dancing, laughing. She should
have married him!

I remember thinking how absolutely crazy the whole
situation was. How could my mother stand by and watch her
second daughter get married at such a young age? How
could my father think this was a good idea just because he
caught her sneaking around with a guy? How could all the
other adults stand by and do nothing? Once I heard the news,
I went back home from Columbus, Ohio, and my VISTA

29

volunteering to talk with my sister and try to change her mind. I was too late. That was the very day she got married. Every once in awhile I wonder if my father chose that day because he knew I was coming and might try to change Christine's mind. By the time I arrived from Kennedy Airport in New York and took the Connecticut Limousine to Bridgeport, my sister was a married teenager. I didn't know this when I arrived. I asked my mother where Christine was but she wouldn't say. I waited and soon enough she arrived, forever changed. I was pissed but there was nothing I could do; there was no way to undo the damage.

Well, I'll never forget The Day. They had everything worked out, where, when we would be married. Theo's brother was going to be in town. (He worked on the ships too, as an engineer.) They thought this was a good time and he would be a good witness to the marriage. I didn't know anything till the morning we were going to drive to Rye, New York to get married by the Justice of the Peace. Thirty years almost to the day I'm writing this – July 27, 1967. I remember I changed my birth date on my certificate from 1951 to 1950 so I would be sixteen – the legal age for marriage.

As if that wasn't enough, my parents also wanted to have a church wedding for me. I didn't want one! Well, I had to wait till I was legally 16 to quit school the following December 26th. I left school regretfully. For five months I went to school secretly married, there was gossip around that I was pregnant, but I wasn't.

Again, I gave in to a church wedding, February 4, 1968, what should have been the happiest day of my life was the worst! All anyone has to do is look at the wedding pictures and they can tell I was not happy. I kept telling myself after this I would leave for good! If my parents wanted me out of the house, then I would go far away. I couldn't help feeling they wanted to get rid of me so they wouldn't have to worry about me anymore. Less problems for them, but what about me?

I now hold some of the black and white wedding photographs Christine mentions. There's one in particular. The bride is looking into our old dining room gilded mirror combing her short hair, which is parted to the left and flipped at the bottom. The bride's left hand holds down her hair as her right hand holds the comb. Her dress is white lace with small buttons and a bow on the upper back. On the bureau directly underneath is my cedar jewelry box on top of my mother's lacework, a carafe of wine, a pack of cigarettes, a tin of tobacco and an ashtray. The bride's eyes are dark with mascara: they have a tragic quality to them, as if they could already see into her future heartaches.

As I stare into my sister's long ago eyes, I notice there's also a painting of the Last Supper reflected in the mirror. It could easily be one of the paint by number canvases our godfather had done. Is the bride looking at the holy gathering and imagining a similar fate for herself? Sacrificed on the cross for the sake of others? I'll never know. I wasn't even there. Maybe I should've made a Dustin Hoffman like scene similar to the one in "The Graduate" when he storms into the church and stops the wedding. Yes, she was already married but I imagined rescuing her anyway. But instead I decided to hide out with my Spanish class. (Mrs. Conchita had arranged for ten of us to go live with families in Mexico during the winter work study program at Goddard College where I went after my VISTA year. The program fell through and we were left on our own. I wandered down to Oaxaca and Puerto Escondido with a girl whose name I don't remember.)

Now I wonder about the series of events that caused relatives and friends to say, "poor Christine, the poor thing, she's had such a hard life," whenever her name was mentioned. Did the damage to my sister's young spirit inevitably bring her to her death thirty-two years later? No, no I say to myself. She had good years, she had three beautiful daughters, she had decades of life, not all of them unhappy. Isn't it similar to my leaving home and the series of unforeseen events that created my future? Perhaps. I'd like to think I had more control in my life than my sister did in hers, but then control was our father's specialty.

I didn't feel in control when I accompanied my sister to the clinic weeks after she discovered she had the virus. My body and mind were on ice as I sat in the passenger seat of the car. Christine was driving and I didn't know what to say and neither did she. I only knew I don't want to lose her so soon after I'd found her. We parked, walked into the clinic and found seats in the waiting room. I looked around and saw faces buried in magazines. There was an AIDS video playing on a large screen television against the opposite wall, but no one was looking at it. A neutral voice spoke of the disease as if he were talking about catching the measles. I couldn't look at the screen either. Christine sat next to me after she checked in. We didn't look like we belonged here. We both looked like we'd rather be shopping.

"Do you want me to come in with you? Or should I wait out here?" I asked, secretly hoping I could get away with not having to hear from a counselor that my sister really had the virus. Maybe there'd been a mistake. I looked around again and saw young, strung-out skinny women.

"I'll go in and ask. Maybe she'll want to see me first and then I can call you in later."

"O.K, I'll wait," I say, relieved that I'd have a few more minutes of denial. Christine's name was called; she walked up, entered the room and closed the door. Good, I could rest a minute. I looked at the television and didn't understand what I was seeing: pictures of white and red blood cells moving wildly inside someone's body. Foreign words like *T-cells, auto immune, deficiencies* popped up and my head spun with the realization that I'd have to learn all about these and how much I didn't want to. I didn't want to. I didn't want to. I didn't want to God- damn it. How come it was me – how come it was my sister – how could it have been My Baby Sister?

Soon Christine came out to get me. I followed her to another, smaller room. A friendly woman told me, "Your sister has HIV which stands for Human Immunodeficiency Virus. She doesn't have AIDS. We recommend she see a doctor and take good care of her body. The virus attacks key cells in the immune system and it may gradually weaken her body's defenses causing her to develop serious illnesses." Her voice was too friendly as she spoke.

"Will my sister get AIDS?" I asked.

"I'm sorry, we just don't know. Your sister could live a long time without getting AIDS. She doesn't have AIDS now but she needs to get a good doctor and start a treatment plan. AZT is a drug that could help."

"Where do we go for this help? I don't know anything about this disease." I said.

"Make another appointment and I'll get you a list of doctors. Do you have health insurance?"

Christine hesitated before she said, "I have some, not much. I don't want anyone to know about this; I'm still working in a flower shop."

"You don't have to tell anyone. Your records should be private."

The words "don't tell, private and fear" jutted out as a warning. Then it suddenly struck me that we were forever branded. We were forever part of the diseased ones, guilty by association. Just like my unknown Greek grandfather who died of influenza. A disease that was highly contagious, spread like wildfire and had brought terror to my mother's family. No one had told us of his quick death, as if he were to blame for dying. Now secrecy enshrouded my sister's disease.

In a few minutes the appointment was over and we got up to leave. Christine didn't say anything and I don't remember what we did for the rest of the day.

Now in the late summer of 2001 I stare at a later photograph to the left of my computer. Christine's picture is in an oval ornate wooden frame. It's a mournful pose as her right hand holds up the left side of her face. We're visiting my girlfriend Sherry and Christine's sitting in an old rocker next to the window. She's wearing a long turquoise sweater and black velvet pants: matching outfits we'd bought together, only my sweater is maroon. Her hair is shoulder length and she has wistful bangs and fluffy hair. Her left hand is between her crossed legs as if for warmth. She stares out at me then as the photographer and me now as the writer. Waiting. Waiting as if to say, "What next? What will you do with me now?"

The picture is not one Christine liked of herself but then she usually hated having her picture taken, unlike my mother and I who are always ready for a pose and a smile. "Don't take my picture, she'd say." I don't feel like it. Don't make me smile when I don't want to. Don't make me look at you." Usually I'd ignore her pleas and take the picture anyway.

Now I wonder what she was thinking in that rocking chair. There was a deep part of my sister that I don't think any one ever knew. She kept herself well hidden behind her half smiles and sullen looks. Was the silence something she had control over? I'm not sure she herself knew. Christine didn't ever have the luxury of unlimited free time to discover what she wanted in life.

Figuring things out was always important to me. I suppose that's why religion didn't have much appeal – everything was already figured out. I had enough questions to fill a lifetime. Are we really being punished for our sins when bad things happen to us? Are we really meant to be happy? Is that possible? Why are we born into this life now? What's the meaning of my life?

Sometimes Christine would ask, "Why do I have this disease? Why did God give it to me? Have I been such a horrible person that I have to be punished this way?" I didn't know what to say besides, "No, no you're not being punished. I don't know why you have it. It's not anything you did; it's not your fault, it's not your fault." In the beginning of her virus I remember wanting to hurt Sal, her adoring boyfriend turned jerk. I wanted to slap him around and scream in his face. "You gave my sister a death sentence! Didn't you think about that when you were shooting up? Didn't you think about the danger you were bringing to yourself and her?" Soon after her diagnosis she stopped saying his name. From then on when she had to say something about her former lover she'd say *He* or *Him* in a swift exhale, brushing aside anything they might have meant to each other. A year later in the spring of 1992 he was dead.

Christine didn't talk about her feelings towards him. I figured they were tortured. She once thought he was her great love, the love she had chosen on her own, the love he too felt for her. I could tell the way they both hung on each other, he with his rough welder's arm over her shoulders and she with her arm around his waist. They both had dark curly hair, they both were short and they both were camera shy. They made a handsome couple.

After the divorce Christine's three girls moved in with them. He bought a house with a big yard, big enough for Christine to have a garden full of tomatoes, big enough for everyone to live in. But the house wasn't big enough to keep misery from finding them. She saw him several times before he died.

What really hurt me was that he never said he was sorry. His only words to me about it was, "How is your AIDS?" He was really far-gone then, living with his parents. Toward the end I remember going to visit him, sitting at the kitchen table and I started to cry uncontrollably when I saw how weak and frail and awful he looked. His parents said I shouldn't do that.

His mother blamed Christine for her son's AIDS. Somehow she had turned into the villain. Italian mothers must be similar to Greek mothers; they can't imagine their sons being at fault for anything that goes wrong in their lives, someone else, something else must be to blame for their misfortune.

At Sal's wake my nieces went to pay their respects. Christine didn't go, fearful of a scene with his family. But my middle niece Tina provided one anyway. She screamed at her older sister Adriana who'd aligned herself with the Italian family, "This guy's killing our mother! How could you stand with them and not with us?" Friends dragged Tina out of the funeral parlor. This embarrassed my sister when she told me the story but secretly I thought maybe she was proud that her daughter had spoken for the mother.

I remember the great sorrow I felt over Adriana's defection. The great sorrow I still feel. It's the one great thing my sister wanted and it's the one great thing I couldn't give her, the gift of her eldest daughter's return.

It's not unlike the return of my eldest, when I finally met my unknown adult birth daughter. It was such a relief; how could I not provide a similar reunion for my sister? How could I not talk her eldest into returning? For years I wrote and I phoned. "Your mom needs you, your mom wants to see you, after she's gone it'll be too late; you'll regret this later." It didn't do any good.

Eventually we lost our once close relationship. Adriana gave me an ultimatum: I could remain her aunt and even come to her wedding along with her Yiayia, my mother, but only on one condition: I couldn't ever speak of her mother, my sister. I couldn't ever try and change her mind. I immediately shouted back, "How are my mother and I supposed to go to your wedding when the rest of the family is uninvited? How can we have a good time knowing your mother and sisters are sitting at home?" I refused and my mother refused because I did.

Now I wonder what made Adriana so rigid. Whenever I'd ask she'd say, "She was a lousy mother, she was never there for me and she was terrible."

"What was so awful that she can't be forgiven? Why can't you talk it out with her? How can you forgive your father but not your mother? How can you let her die without saying good-bye?" I only got, "I don't want to talk about it." Adriana's heart had shut out her mother and her sisters who had always aligned themselves with their mother. I suppose Adriana might think of herself as the smart one who got away.

I remember the last visit my sister made to us in Chicago, four months before her death. She was very frail, but her doctor said she could travel. Christine wanted to see our remodeled rooms and new wood floors and she wanted to see her daughter Tina's new home in Las Vegas. I traveled to Connecticut and brought her back with me. She stayed several days and then flew on her own to her daughter. She returned a week later and stayed the weekend before going back to Connecticut. We were all aware this was her last trip; her body was caving in on itself. I brought her to Unity church. I rushed her that morning so we could make the nine a.m. service but her one speed was slow so I shut my mouth and waited. We got into the car and five minutes later we were in the parking lot of the church. We walked slowly up the steps, my arm locked in with hers.

"Where should we sit? Maybe the back row in case you have to go to the bathroom, what do you think?" I said anxious to get her seated and out of the crowd gathering at the door.

"I'll follow you – go ahead. I'm right behind you," she said quietly.

I led us to the back row up against the windows and near the heat. I wanted Christine to feel what I felt, to love this room, this congregation, this minister and this service as much as I did.

It's love I felt for this space that I had discovered in the winter of 1996. My neighbor had brought me with her. I was desperate to make a spiritual connection. I was convinced I wouldn't like it but I went anyway. As soon as we entered the wide-open room filled with windows and light I felt an excitable energy vibrating with warm voices, laughter, and sunshine. It looked like a party room, so unlike the solemn Greek and Romanian Churches we had grown up in. I immediately felt invited. My neighbor guided me to a seat in the middle of the room and I sat and watched the others around me. There were young people with children; middle- aged people like me and older people. Happy groups of people holding hands, short- haired women rubbing each other's shoulders, men laughing, children on laps. I looked at white, black, and Asian faces. I was comforted by the mix; I could easily fit in here. When the service began we stood and the Lord's Prayer was sung in a beautiful, slow melodic tone. I started to cry, but forced myself to stop. I didn't know why I was crying. I'd only known that if I'd started I wouldn't have stopped.

On this Sunday with Christine I wanted her to be comforted like I'd been comforted and then maybe her sullen face would brighten. (I realize now it's something I tried to do often, make her smile, laugh, be happy to be alive.) I sat and couldn't help looking over at her every few minutes to measure her reaction to the Lord's Prayer, the meditation, the singing and the sermon. At the beginning of the service the minister asked if anyone was there for the first time and I raised my hand towards Christine. A woman came over and handed her a white carnation and a brochure. Christine's face was unreadable, except when they were singing; she smiled then. She had always liked the singing. (Later she told me her favorite songs were "Dust in the Wind" by Guns N' Roses and "The Heart of the Matter" by Don Henley. We played both at her funeral.) I was a bundle of nerves and when it came time to relax for meditation, I couldn't do it. I worried over what she might be meditating about. Did she pray for a quick death? A slow death? No death? Did she pray for an afterlife? Or was it as simple as wishing for a cup of coffee?

"So what did you think?" I said as I put my face close to hers when it was over.

"I liked it, the music especially, and the minister is funny. I gotta use the bathroom. Take me to the bathroom."

"I'll walk you over there. It's just across the hall." I took her left elbow and we waited with the rest of the congregation filing out of the room. On the way I met Mary, who was in my Toastmaster's group that also met there. It was there that I practice my stories out loud. It was there at Unity I had learned to speak of my sister's disease.

"This is my sister," I said to her. "She's visiting from out of town." There was a slight hesitation before she spoke. I wondered what she thought as she stared at me and then at my sister's ravaged face and fallen body. Did she remember any of the stories I'd read about my sister to the group? Did she hook the story with the face in front of her?

"Nice to meet you. Excuse me but I have to rush out and find my friend before she leaves." Mary turned quickly before my sister could get out a "hi."

I was disappointed; I wanted Christine to feel welcome. After the bathroom we went downstairs for coffee. I don't remember having seen anyone else I knew there. We went to the bookstore to get a free tape of the day's sermon. Weeks and months later I was glad she'd seen what I've been talking about for years. I prayed she could imagine herself in such a place also. I prayed she could imagine an inviting community that would take her in. I prayed she would find comfort in the energy around her as she prepared for the journey ahead. Suddenly it struck me that maybe Christine hadn't wanted any of that because her comfort had lain simply in having me next to her. Maybe where we were hadn't really mattered and I hadn't needed to control the time we had together.

Just now the word control doesn't look right as I type it. I reach over for the dictionary behind the printer and see there are six different meanings for this word. It's the fourth meaning: "to exercise authority over; direct; command," which I associate with my father. I see the sixth meaning could easily apply to my mother: "to hold back; curb; restrain (control your grief). They seem to be opposites – like my parents.

Certainly I'm more like my father than my mother. As the oldest I like to command and direct. Christine was more like my mother, stuffing tears and dreams in a dark spot in the pit of her stomach. My older brother Jimmy is more like me and my younger brother Tas is more like Christine. Was this pre-destined when our names were given to us: my brother and I receiving our father's parents names and my sister and brother receiving our mother's parents names? I resist the easiness of this explanation. Certainly my siblings probably would, too. It seems we're a combination of both their temperaments. But still, it's tempting to have my father claim his two eldest and my mother claim her two youngest.

I remember one time when I told my father off. It was his eightieth birthday, a year before his death and three years before Christine's diagnosis. I'd flown from Chicago so we could take him out to dinner. There was some screw-up with rides and we were late getting to my folks' house. Maybe I was already there waiting for my sister and brothers. Anyway my dad was fuming, roaming, cursing under his breath. I knew by his half clenched teeth and his vile energy that he was bad off. It was past six o'clock and he hadn't eaten. He also hated waiting and hated being late. (All of these things I also hate.) So they were an hour late. They walk in and I said, "Oh, let's go so we can eat. We've picked a nice seafood restaurant."

We watched my father roam from room to room like a caged animal. We all sat down in the living room waiting for him to say or do something.

"It's too late – it's too late to go out. Where have you all been God damn it?" He turned to face us and his arms were over his head ready to strike. "Where have you been when I'm here waiting for you? Forget it – I don't want to go out now – it's too late." Suddenly he put his arms down and turned towards the hall closet and started grabbing shirts off the hangers. "There's nothing clean, I can't find a damn shirt to wear! Where are all my shirts? He grabbed a white shirt and began tearing the sleeves and collar with large swinging motions. The pieces lay on the floor next to him.

The five of us sat frozen on the couch. My mom was between us for protection. I stared at the buttons on the sleeves and they became small eyes searching for a spot to rest. Had this guy lost all of his marbles? I looked up at my father and his eyes were hungry with fire. His mouth was open and his tongue was bright red. He yelled *Glara, Glara* or "crazy woman, crazy woman" at my mother who had bent her head into her apron. It must have been her fault that he couldn't find a shirt to wear. We watched in silence, praying this would not last long.

Suddenly something in me snapped. I couldn't take the silence. Who did this guy think he was? He was acting like an idiot, father or no father. Before I could think about what to say or how to say it I blurted out, "Pop why are you ripping up your shirt? Why can't we just go out now that everyone's here? Why are you yelling at mom? Put on any shirt and let's go!" The last thing I wanted to do was go out with this guy, but there's no way any of us could get out of it. It was his birthday

There was silence. Then there was "Shush, shush, shush," aimed my way by my mom and siblings. Were they afraid he was going to blow? There was more silence. He didn't say anything, but suddenly turned and walked into the kitchen, away from us.

"Why did you make him madder? Why didn't you just be quiet?" Jimmy said. He couldn't believe I had yelled at our father like my father yelled at my mother.

"He's acting stupid. Are we just going to sit and watch him rip clothes? I thought we were going out to eat." I knew I'd crossed the line. "Screw this, I'm an adult for God sakes. I don't take this from anyone. I gotta take it from him? No sir."

There was more silence. Someone went into the kitchen to get him. Eventually he went back in the closet and found a clean, un-torn shirt. We went to the restaurant. It was a fancy place. At least it wasn't a diner. We ordered fresh shrimp, scallops and calamari, except for my dad - he ordered a hot dog. I don't remember singing happy birthday to him later when the cake arrived, but we must have said something.

The next morning I approached him at the kitchen table. "Pop, I hate the yelling, the swearing, the mean words towards Mom, I can't take it anymore."

"Respect your father and don't yell back to your father. I'm your father, always remember that." I looked around; others had just walked into the kitchen and then quickly walked out. I didn't know what else to say.

Now, I suddenly remember this was also the time he gave each of us a check for thousands of dollars and said, "I made money the hard way for the four of you. Don't spend on foolish things. Save as much as you can." (Christine bought her first- ever new, black car that she'd have for the rest of her life. I paid bills, bought a futon bed and had some of my brother's paintings framed. I don't know what my brothers did with their money.)

Now again, it strikes me that our Dad was like a kid who couldn't have his goody when he wanted it. He wanted it at a particular time or not at all. (On the first page of his autobiography, I had helped him with, he wrote of his first memory, "One summer day, we had a school party, and everyone got a bag of candy. On the way from school, going home happy, a teenage boy approached me and grabbed my fancy bag of candy. I started to cry. And that was it. The boy disappeared." It felt as if his happiness had vanished after that.)

I've got that stubbornness too. If things don't go the way I plan, I think they're going badly. Why is it so hard to let things happen the way they were meant to happen? Maybe it's letting go that's so difficult after a lifetime of hanging on to the illusion of being in control. It's the not knowing that's so terrifying. Or maybe it's not having the faith to know that all will unfold in due time.

I do know my sister learned she wasn't in control early in her life. She learned not to hang on to the illusion and maybe that's what allowed her to live her last years with a dignity and grace I'm not sure I possess.

Until I Sleep

We never spoke my parents' language. I was sorry about that. We could understand what they were saying most of the time, but couldn't speak it. My father also spoke about six or seven other languages. My parents were not affectionate people; an occasional peck on the cheek was all I got. I never really felt loved by them, yet they probably did in their own way.

I've just returned from a fourth trip this year to visit my mom in a Connecticut nursing home. My heart opens and closes at her slow loss of body, mind, and spirit. So unlike my dad, who took everything he could take with him. So unlike Christine, who left everything behind so she could travel into the next life with comfort. Have we always spoken a different language, unable to translate our emotions into words? Did that deep well between feeling and understanding help create our individual miseries? I love to play with words just like our father loved to play with languages.

How will I end up? Where will I breathe my last breath? My mom is terrified of dying alone. Earlier, when she still had her apartment, a visiting nurse said what a nice thing it'd be to die quietly in one's bed. My mother looked at her as if she were nuts. She didn't say anything but her look implied, "Yeah lady, maybe for you but not for me. I'm not dying alone in my sleep."

It was when she could no longer live alone that my mom wanted me to say, "Well, mom come live with us.

Come to Chicago." I didn't say it then, although I had said it another time. No, no she had said then, her boys, her church, she couldn't leave them. Later she was scared and wanted me to take her away. But by then I could see how it would never have worked. I could see how she would be so needy, so dependent on me and only me. I would have grown angrier and been nasty to her and to the kids and Michael. Life would have turned into a "full -blown catastrophe" just like Zorba the Greek had predicted in his movie of the same name.

Now I wonder, will my children take me in? Certainly I don't expect it. Don't even want it. I imagine being on my own with or without a partner by the ocean and plenty of lifelong friends nearby. We'll take care of each other in our old age. Yes, it's a romantic notion, but one I still maintain.

It's this romantic notion I tried to get Christine to believe in too. I remember giving her the popular novel *Talk Before Sleep*, by Elizabeth Berg, about a dying woman surrounded by loving friends who feed, talk to and nurture her. I wanted her to get used to the idea of dying and how it didn't have to be such a lonely experience. Christine read the book, but didn't say much. If she had talked it would have meant she was getting used to the idea of not being around forever. It would have meant she could see the value in having friends. It would have meant I wouldn't have to work so hard.

Now I see it was me I was really worried about. How was I going to manage without her? How was the future going to unfold? How was I going to manage my own death? Christine was never a talkative person. Why didn't I understand or respect her silence?

Maybe I really did understand what her silence meant. Did I understand but not accept the depression, the disappointments, and the hardships in her life? Or did I not understand and accept the mystery that would always enshroud her, the deep mystery that lives within each one of us?

44

A part of me wants to blame her for not being more assertive, for not deciding what she wanted and then taking steps to get there. Does that take a certainty my sister didn't possess until later in life? Now as I re-read her journal, I'm reminded of just how hard her teenage life was.

I remember being torn between the Greek and American cultures – since Theo was very Greek that's the way we lived – Greek women "should stay home" and tend to the home. That's what my mother did, so I figured, "I'll do the same."

I got pregnant and had my first daughter "Adriana" (a name I picked because I liked it) on Jan. 6,1969, the year I should have graduated with my class.

Theo got involved with Greek friends, restaurant owners that promised him excellent salaries; and he did do very well financially. He knew his job and was very good with customers; everybody liked him. He would call everyone his friend! After awhile the novelty in Theo wore off. I realized that he wasn't an honest person. We never left Connecticut like he promised. He got too involved with his friends and didn't want to leave.

Soon after I got pregnant again and had my 2nd daughter Tina, named her after me, on May 16, 1970.

Theo always worked nights. He was a hard worker - he had the 7 p.m. to 7 a.m. shift at a local diner.

He was great with the girls, always laughing and playing with them. I thought, "how nice," since I never knew that either in my life. His job was playing with them, not changing diapers; that was my job.

He was a joker all right. It got to the point where he took absolutely nothing seriously. Money was no object. He started getting into heavy debts; he was addicted to gambling and sometimes he would not come home for days.

I dreaded payday, praying he would come home. Many times he didn't. There were no casinos in those days. He liked to play cards, at friend's houses or the Greek coffee house, as it was called.

After awhile he wanted to buy the coffee house and my father helped him! To me, it was like an alcoholic buying a bar. I was furious at my father. All my father could see was dollar signs- the place did rake in tons of money- but what good was it, Theo would sit down and gamble the money away?

I pleaded with him many times to buy a small diner or luncheonette where we both could work. But he thought he could do much better at the coffee house.

He thought he was Mr. "Hot Shit." He even traded the '67 Camaro my father bought us for a brand new silver Chevelle – without even telling me- he just drove it into the driveway one day. I loved my Camaro but never got a chance to drive it. I didn't get my license 'til I was 20.

Why did I get to leave and not my sister? Why did someone have to stay behind? Aren't I the one that's left behind after all? Was my freedom gained at my sister's expense? Is my freedom like having to extract a bride price in an arranged marriage? Someone was going to have to pay.

Growing up I had thought I was the smart one who would get away. I don't remember when this feeling came to me; I only remember it growing stronger as I got older. And yet, could I really get away from what was locked in my heart? Could I really leave eighteen years of my life behind? All the back and forth trips to my father, then my sister, and now to my mother leave me wondering. What was I hoping, what am I hoping for still? To be considered the good daughter, the good sister, the smart one, maybe even to be considered the one who's right. My father never doubted he was right. He told us so every chance he got. "Listen to me; I know what's right. Don't listen to me and you're wrong." There were only two sides in my father's heart: his side and everyone else's.

Now I know writing this book has helped me to see my sister, see me and see the events of our lives in a clearer light. In a light that doesn't cast blame or guilt.

I also know I will never be a good enough daughter. The title of a recent memoir grabs my attention, *The Bad Daughter*. The author leaves home to find a life of her own and never returns, not even when her mother is dying. The author is young and I don't much care for the book, but it reminds me of my oldest niece, Adriana, and how she could have written a similar story. For them, nothing will ever be good enough.

Christine lived a good enough eight years with the virus: 3 years with HIV and 5 years with AIDS. A sudden death would not have been good enough. I'm afraid of the lack of preparation – the transition time needed to go from being to non-being. Christine faced the transition with great dignity. There's a part of me that's tempted to say, "fuck it" to pain and screw ups – I don't look at it as a challenge, a puzzle to be worked out. Christine did. She always found a way to live, to work and to buy things for her daughters. She always dragged herself to the bathroom to throw up, to spit up and to clean herself up. I'd be tempted to do it all in bed. Christine kept going long beyond the point anyone thought she would. Weeks before she died I was helping her to the bathroom at Hospice, and she'd combed her hair and was putting on lipstick. I was praying she didn't look too closely into the mirror.

"Connie, what's this stuff on my face?" she said. "Do you think it's something else to worry about?"

My heart jumped up to my throat as I thought, you're dying for Christ's sake. Your body is shot; it's probably some kind of cancerous growth.

Out loud I said, "It's probably a side effect from the medicine. It'll go away, don't worry about it."

"Well I'm going to ask the nurse if there's something she can do for it. Maybe there's an ointment or cream I can use." Christine looked away from the mirror.

Maybe she believed me, maybe she didn't, but her hand rested comfortably on mine as I took her back to bed in a room she shared with no one.

Just now the phone rings next to the computer. I pick it up on the second ring. Maybe it's something important, something that will force me to stop writing, a temptation that often lurks quietly beside me like an impatient child: Stop now, Mom and come out and play. Stop, stop working and sit on the floor with me. Stop, stop and pay attention to me.

It's my friend Deb who lives down the alley. After our hellos I say, "I'm in the middle of writing. You know about Christine. I'm not sure how to keep going – the pieces are so overwhelming." Deb is one of the few people I've shared my writing worries with – not that she's a writer-she's a painter, a nurse and my walking buddy. Deb's got two sisters, one older and one younger- both still alive. She's also one of several people who has read my first manuscript, *It's All Greek to Me.*

(Months before Christine's death, I had mentioned this title to her and she had laughed, "Yeah, being Greek didn't help us figure out a damn thing!)

"Just keep writing; Christine will help you. Why else would she leave her journals behind? She could've thrown them out."

"I can't imagine her doing that, just like I can't imagine throwing out any of my journals – I keep my old appointment calendars and address books for God's sake!" We laugh and I wonder why I value paper, books and photographs more than clothes, jewelry or furniture. Am I hidden between neatly bound sheets of paper? I continue talking,

"She should've never gotten AIDS. Why her, she didn't fuck around with strangers." I stop at the word strangers and remember my mom's warning, "Don't tell family secrets to strangers!" But what happens when your parents and siblings become the real strangers?

"Your sister was brave – that's the part you have to tell. Just how brave she was once she found out she had the

48

virus. I don't know how I could bear to live with death so close by."

Just then I remember a mother I saw on television years ago, rushing out for ice cream, getting into a fatal car accident and never returning. My heart still jumps at the thought: Wait! It was just ice cream she was going after; she can't die because she wanted dessert for her family can she?

"Nothing makes the kind of sense we're looking for, nothing can explain why someone dies and another lives. Nothing can explain the suffering of those left behind. I'm afraid of that kind of suffering for myself." Deb says.

"Then what am I doing? I always thought writing could bring meaning to our chaotic lives. I always thought words were the way out of pain." A sudden heavy lump plops like a gray rock into my heart.

"Don't give up, you have to tell the story the best way you know how. I wish I could say the same for my painting. I give up too easily most days. The unfinished canvas waits for me to say, ' Okay let me pick up my brush and make it breathe.' The temptation to mop the floor or clean the toilets often wins."

"Yeah, I was just thinking your phone call might be a legitimate distraction, something that would force me to stop." I say.

"I know that feeling. I admire your ability to keep at it. Hey, if it's a decent weekend, let's walk. We shouldn't stop because of the cold. We can bundle up in layers. As long as we keep moving, we'll be all right."

We say our good-byes and I hang up the phone. Writing is such a lonely affair. Sometimes I wish I didn't have this nagging urge to make sense of my life with words. At other times I only wish the words would come easier.

Several years earlier I was searching for words as I held onto Christine and hoped for a distraction from her misery. She'd just gotten out of Yale New Haven's hospital after having had surgery to remove polyps in her throat. We were waiting for her morphine prescription at a nearby

49

pharmacy. It was frigid outside and I asked Christine if she wanted to browse around in the Yale co-op bookstore next door. We had twenty-five minutes and she said yes. I held the door open with my left hand and used my right to clutch my sister's elbow. Christine was fragile and doped up; I don't remember what else was wrong with her. There were so many ailments by then: stomach viruses, numbing and swelling of feet, extreme itching, diarrhea, throwing up, hacking coughs, migraine headaches, extreme fatigue and wasting away.

I looked around and saw the store was almost empty: two employees at the register talking and several students browsing through the used textbook shelves. There was a table by the entrance with the latest New York Times bestsellers at ten percent off the regular price, still no bargain. Nothing caught my eyes as I followed Christine. She shuffled between the aisles and pretended to be all right.

"Do you want to go back and wait in the car?" I asked.

"I'm O.K, Let's just walk around."

I led her to the back of the store and found a sale table. Our eyes lit up as we saw the word "sale." Maybe there'd be some good junk we could load up on. There was an odd assortment of stuff; Van Husen men's white dress shirts originally $38.00 now only what, $1.00! art calendars, $1.00, hair scrunchies, $1.00, danskin tights, $1.00!

We turned toward each other and smiled as our hands started sifting through for sizes and colors. I looked for Danskin tights that might fit and Christine began to load up on gifts.

"What would Jason like?" she asked.

"How about this Batman flashlight?"

I stood close in case she needed to lean into me. I turned left and looked into her face. There was nothing written on it.

"Are you getting tired, should we leave now? I asked again.

"I want to stand, I've been lying in bed for days"

What was I doing shopping while my sister waited for her morphine? Maybe I should have insisted on our waiting in the car. Just then Christine turned to me and said,

"Connie, let's buy a bunch of these calendars," as if she could buy time for others to mark up with important dates.

We spent the next ten minutes picking out the best stuff; we loaded our arms with all the unexpected loot. Christine took all the hair scrunchies for our daughters. Before the drugs she used to like to wear these on her thick long hair. I looked over at her and wanted to cry at the thin strands on her head. I watched her doing something so ordinary in an extraordinary body. Was it OK to shop now? Maybe we should be doing something more important.

I didn't know what that was. I thought about who might want a calendar in March. Everyone had already stocked up. What was left would be thrown out with the trash.

Christine grabbed seven calendars and I took the remaining two. She smiled and for a few minutes she'd gotten at least nine more months.

In fact, she had those nine months plus fifteen more. There would be more trips to the hospital and emergency room. There would be more visits from Chicago, each time wondering whether it would be the last, each time wanting the waiting to end; each time wanting the waiting to go on forever.

Christine is gone and the distance is now an eternity. She was once afraid of being left behind. Now she's the one leading and I'm the one forced to tag along. It's an idea that took a long while to get used to. Wasn't I supposed to go – wasn't I supposed to die - before my sister or my brothers? How was Christine going to manage without me?

I don't know if she ever cried over this. I don't know if she ever saw the unfairness of it. I do know she didn't express anger or bitterness to me that I would live and she wouldn't. I do know if I were in her shoes I'd be fighting

51

mad. So maybe the question was really, How were we going to manage without Christine?

Years earlier, I had been the one to tell my brothers and mother. In the early nineties the virus was slowly transforming from a gay disease into a drug disease and clean needle exchange programs were being debated. Many thought giving drug addicts clean needles supported their habit. Others thought drug addicts were going to shoot up anyway so protect them and others from getting HIV with a dirty needle. Not much was said about the sex partners of drug addicts. Not much was said about the rapid rise in women being infected by their partner's habit or sexuality.

I told my brothers not long after the diagnosis. I told my mom much later. I didn't know what to expect. I only knew I didn't want hysterics. Or maybe I did. Maybe I wanted wailing and sobbing over the tragedy of an early death. I didn't get it though. I chose a neutral time when I was alone with my brothers at my mom's house to tell them. Life was not going well for them either.

"I have something to say about Christine. You know she's not being feeling well for a long time."

"How come? What's the matter with her?" Jim said." Is it some kind of cancer?"

"No it's not cancer, I wish it was."

"Is it a disease she got from that nut case she's been with?" Tas said.

"Christine has the HIV virus. She'll probably get AIDS – that's what Sal has."

"That jerk, I hope he rots in hell. He was nuts right from the beginning. I knew he was no good. I hope he suffers and rots." Jim said.

"He'll die soon enough. Christine may get to live a long while with these new medicines. It's all experimental - nobody knows anything for sure." I said sounding like I was talking about someone other than our sister.

"Shit, why poor Christine? Why her and not some asshole who screws guys?" Tas said.

There was no answer to the why question. My brothers didn't know what to do except badmouth the Italian. I couldn't imagine what my father would have done if he were alive. Sometimes I'd fantasized the three of them taking on the Italians, kicking their asses and making them take back the virus. "Here assholes. Christine doesn't need this; take it and shoot it back up your bloodsucking veins!"

A year after her HIV diagnosis Christine moved into a 3-bedroom condo on Hemlock Road with my mom and two of her daughters. My mom had sold the house she lived in with my dad and bought the condo. The second day of the move I called Christine and she was in a panic.

"It's a mistake, the move is a mistake. It's not going to work out. How could I have thought I could live with that woman? I can't live with Mom. What made me think I could? It's a mistake, oh God it's a big mistake."

"Christine, the place sounds beautiful. You've got your bedroom upstairs with your own bath and Mom's downstairs. There's room for you and the girls and mom." I was mad at my sister for putting a damper so quickly on this move. I was relieved to have them both "settled" into nice living quarters with lots of space and sunlight, so unlike what they'd each been living in. Also it didn't hurt that it took the pressure off of me to take care of Mom.

Christine was right; it didn't work. Her health deteriorated and she hated having to share a kitchen and living room with her mother. My mom didn't know what was wrong with her daughter and she was afraid to press after Christine would say, "I'm all right just a little sick. Just leave me alone." Christine couldn't tell our mother what was wrong with her. I'm not sure why. Was she afraid our mom would see it as punishment for divorcing her beloved son-in-law and living with an Italian? Would our mom blame her for her illness? During the four years they lived in the condo no one told my mom. For many years we all wanted to believe that Christine would get better, especially in the beginning. All she had to do was find the right drug, the right diet or the right medical interventions. Finally, after they had gotten separate apartments and Christine was getting worse instead of better, I asked if she wanted me tell our mother.

"I don't care," she said, "I just don't want her to keep bugging me. I don't want to have to worry about her too."

"We can't keep it from her any longer. I'll tell her soon." I said.

"OK but tell her I don't want to talk with her about it. I especially don't want to hear all the religious stuff about saving my soul and being sorry for my sins and all that."

"All right. I don't know how she's going to take it. But I'll tell her you have the virus, that you're on medication and have a good doctor." Secretly I was afraid Mom might have a heart attack and I wouldn't know what to do to save her. (She'd already had an attack years earlier, soon after my father died.) I needn't have worried; she didn't express much emotion when I told her. Maybe she already knew something was very wrong. Maybe she wasn't as fragile as we liked to portray her. I too was nonchalant; I could have been talking about the common cold. I remember feeling disappointed; I wanted us to look into each other's eyes and cry and cry over this tragedy. I wanted to connect with this woman who was my mother. I wanted her to hold me and to tell me it was going to be all right. I certainly didn't act like that's what I longed for, but then I'm my mother's daughter after all.

Now I realize I shouldn't have been surprised. My mom doesn't show her emotions. At her husband's funeral, I didn't see a tear; nor at her sisters', nor her mother's. It's just that I kept thinking death is different. Death has got to make people act differently. The death of a daughter has got to be different. If nothing else: death should rattle the heart. If nothing else the death of my sister has left a deep well of loneliness that hungers for recognition and affection from those I love.

Drug Journal Companion

Feb. 91 – Diagnosed HIV positive at Women's Health Services – State Street- New Haven, CT.
Holy Shit!
Went to Yale – Nathan Smith Clinic & started taking the drug AZT.
So many mixed emotions! Anger is the most powerful – I never did drugs! I never abused alcohol – I wasn't a slut! Why Me God? Haven't I suffered enough in my life? It's not fair! I always took care of myself, never even smoked cigarettes. AIDS is something other people get- <u>not me.</u>

I sip my coffee and look at my e-mails. Nothing new. Is there someone I need to write and have forgotten about? I can't remember. Suddenly I remember the dirty laundry. I jump up from the chair and run upstairs to get the overflowing basket and bring it to the basement. I sort the darks and whites and put the darks in the washer first. Then I smell our cat Sonny's litter box nearby and I stoop over to clean out the clumps of poop. Sonny's sister died years ago when they were both kittens. We had gotten to thinking they'd keep each other company. When Moony died we buried her in the backyard with a ceremony full of flowers, candles and incense. It was the first death for Jason and Mika. "Mom, won't we ever see her again? Won't Sonny be lonely now?" Oh, yes, I said all the right things: Mooney's in heaven. She can see us we just can't see her. Don't worry; we'll keep Sonny company so he won't feel lonely.

Now I wonder if Christine's in heaven looking down on us and if the loneliness will ever disappear. Moony was the playful one and my favorite. I've never warmed up to her brother who seems to be living forever.

Christine's cat, Shag, kept her company for years. He was large, long- haired, and slow, as if he had all the time in the world. Towards the end she also had her grandchild. In March of 1998 on a yellow legal sized pad she wrote,

> *Shag Meister T. Sassafras*
> *My Cat, My Guardian Angel, My friend.*
> *He's beautiful, so good, so well behaved.*
> *Content, like my Mikey.*
> *They don't care that I have AIDS.*
> *They don't care that I look ugly as hell.*
> *They still love me.*
> *Mikey hugs and kisses me.*
> *He loves me anyway.*

Had Christine felt unloved by the rest of us? Had she sensed a pulling away from her family but not from the old cat and the young boy who hadn't imagined a world without her?

Back upstairs I pick up my coffee. It's ice cold. I step into the kitchen and put the cardboard cup in the microwave to heat up. I bring it to the back room.

I close my eyes and fold my hands over the keyboard and hum my favorite Unity song: "Our thoughts are prayers and we are always praying, our thoughts are prayers so think of what you're saying. Seek a higher consciousness, a state of peacefulness and know that God, and know that God is always there. And every thought and every thought becomes a prayer." What if our obsessive daily thoughts are really small prayers? The universe must be teeming with shopping lists, needless worries and thoughts spinning out of control. Slowly the litter box, the laundry and cold coffee recede into the folds of my mind. I enter a clear space, open my eyes and pick up Christine's journal.

Today I begin the work of transcribing Christine's drug journal into the computer. This gray journal sat by her bedside for almost eight years and in it she recorded her diagnosis, her symptoms, her medications, her hospitalizations.

Until recently I thought I was going to write this book with Christine's doctor. I figured she'd take care of the medical part and my hands would be clean of that mess, the physical suffering, the numerous visits to the emergency room, and the countless bottles of pills.

This journal isn't one of the many I'd given her over the years. It's a plain cheap gray marbled notebook 5½ x 8½ sized pages – so unlike the expensive-artistic ones I'd given her that will forever remain blank. Suddenly I wonder what's happened to those fancy journals. Did Christine see them as another big sister idea she had no desire to fulfill? Did she recycle them as gifts? Did they eventually get thrown out?

I place the journal on my lap and wait for the words to penetrate through my velveteen pants to my thighs and up around my stomach where I can feel a churning of desires – not only to write this book but to be able to pick up the phone and talk with Christine once again. To reach out and touch her sad face, her thin shoulder, her warm hand, to have a sister who's still alive. I don't know if that desire will ever go away, but maybe when I finish this book some of the churning will subside. I feel a shiver go through both my arms and down into my cold fingers. The coffee cup is empty. I put my hands under my armpits for warmth and then get up to make myself a cup of hot Lipton's tea with spoonfuls of honey and milk. We both preferred milk to lemon in our tea.

As I'm holding the warm cup back at the computer I wonder why Christine decided to keep a record of her drug treatments. Did she imagine it to be a temporary exercise she could stop once she got on the right medication? Did she imagine beating the virus with her determination and strong will? Did writing the dates, the drugs and the side effects, make them more real? Maybe make them more manageable? It's certainly something I would have done.

I count the forty pages she used up – exactly half the journal. The rest of the pages are blank with the last page torn out. Did she use it for scratch paper? Did she write something and then throw it out? Did she mean to leave something more on the last page, words that might explain her long periods of silence, silence I was never much good at interpreting, silence our mother was so good at displaying. Sometimes I wonder if silence isn't a part of growth. Was Christine's silence a sign that she was unhappy, longing for more of everything like our mother? Or was it a sign that she was happy, content to have others around her without a need for words? I remember once she'd entered Hospice I asked her if she wanted me to bring her journal and she said no, no it was too late for that.

Now I wish I had asked her what she meant. Did she mean she was out of time and there was no use recording any longer? Or did she mean the writing had failed in keeping her alive and therefore was useless? Don't we write mainly to stay alive? Don't I think I'll live longer if I keep writing? How could I die before completing a book? Whenever I hear of such things I shudder at the injustice of it. What happens to all those unfinished works? The universe is cluttered with pages floating, unhindered by binders, clasps or rubber bands.

I'll never forget the first time I met Christine's doctor, Nancy Angoff, in 1993. We were at the Yale clinic in New Haven, Connecticut where Christine was to spend many hours over the next six years. It was the clinic I accompanied her to whenever I was in town. On this first visit, I was a basket case; you'd have thought I was the one with AIDS. The waiting room was small and impersonal. The U-shaped wall couch was worn and the center coffee table littered with old magazines. The room was dim and a television was turned on to a soap opera. I wanted to turn it off. If life is reduced to the stupid gestures of pretty people, what was the point of living? Besides, no one was watching. Several starved looking bodies sat and leaned sideways with their eyes closed. My immediate response was to turn around and walk out, but I couldn't. Christine was already at the check-in desk. I followed her and soon we sat and waited to be called.

"You'll like Dr. Angoff," Christine said. "She's really nice. She takes her time with me and makes sure to explain everything so I'll understand. She's never in a hurry with me. I told her about you living in Chicago and coming to visit me; I told her I'd be bringing you."

"She sounds good." I wasn't sure what else to say. All I knew was that it was important I was there, someone to represent the family, to let her doctor know she was not alone. I looked around and hoped to God nobody thought I was the one who was sick. I also hoped no one thought my sister was a drug addict or a prostitute. The few who were in the waiting room with us looked strung out on dope. One of them opened his eyes and said, "Hey, one of you got a cigarette? I could use a cigarette."

I wanted to say, Buddy you're already a fuckin' torch about to ignite, why bother? Instead I said, "We don't smoke. Sorry." I looked over at Christine but she wasn't paying attention.

She still looked all right – I was relieved she looked like the living. This was a couple of years after her initial HIV diagnosis and the disease hadn't yet ravaged her body. Her hair was still long and full. Her weight was decent.

AIDS. When I first heard the word in the mid-eighties I had thought of flesh colored band-aids or aides who helped sick people, like nurse's aides. A part of my mind still thought that – a part of my mind shuffled to accommodate the new meaning that didn't include assistance in any way. It was always a sharp jolt, like those paddles paramedics used to re-start a heart, the shock of remembering the four letters that meant a foreign thing: *Acquired Immune Deficiency Syndrome.*

Soon we were called into the doctor's office. Christine stood and I followed her into the double doors that would take us to the office. She knew right where she was going. Several smiling staff women greet her warmly as she kept walking. How are you doing? they asked.

"I'm living – this is my sister Connie. She's visiting me from Chicago."

I grinned and waved but didn't say anything. I kept walking behind Christine.

An attractive, petite middle- aged woman came to greet us. Was she the doctor? She looked too nice. No scowl, no lab coat, no hurried look in her eyes. As we sat in the office I was struck by her poise and her soft- spoken manner. I felt like a loud immigrant even though I wasn't saying much. Dr. Angoff was wearing an expensive but simple outfit and large silver jewelry complimenting her dark pants and sweater. Her black and gray hair framed her face nicely. Christine and I both had on bulky sweaters and loose pants. I reached up to fluff my wild hair away from my face, but that didn't make me feel more attractive. It was just one of those bad hair days. I concentrated on listening instead of my looks. We introduced ourselves, talked about my flight, the weather, and Chicago for several minutes.

"Your sister is amazing," she said to me. "She's learning so much about her disease and teaching me some things too. There's a lot going on lately with new drug trials. I can't keep up with all of it so she tells me what she'd like more information on and I follow up on it. Right now she is doing fine."

The doctor had a soothing voice. I didn't know what to say. I asked medication and treatment questions but my heart had flown to the fearful place of Christine's probable death even though there was still hope, hope that the virus could be kept in check and my sister could live indefinitely with the disease. I was afraid to ask the questions that couldn't be answered: Will my sister die from this disease doctor? Will I be forced to witness her dying? Will I be forced to witness her death?

In the years ahead the doctor and I became friends. Eventually I called her by her first name. We talked on the phone regularly about the progression of Christine's disease, I sent her books like *Women's Bodies/Women's Wisdom,* and we e-mailed each other often. Eventually we talked about writing a book. I told Christine this several times, but she didn't say much. I suppose I wanted the "go ahead" from her; I wanted my sister to say, "That's great! Let me give you some ideas." At the time I was desperate to show Christine that she'd be loved long after she'd left us, that she wouldn't be forgotten, that through my writing she'd always continue to live. Now I see the desperation was more for me than for her. Wasn't I trying to extend her life through words? Wasn't I making the promise so I could have her life continue through mine?

Two years after Christine's death I met the doctor at the Hyatt in downtown Chicago while she was in town for an AIDS- related conference. The lobby was busy with tourists and conventioneers. I was early so I stood against a glass wall with an earlier manuscript, a legal pad and pen. I watched nicely dressed women and men go up and down the escalator. I glared into faces for signs of emotion – two attractive brunettes descended laughing with bright eyes and an older couple stepped up, careful not to miss the moving stairs. I was anxious to meet Nancy and get our project off the ground. Would she still be agreeable to writing a book together? How would it work? I saw her coming down, a petite and trim woman only several years older than I but looking more a part of the lobby scene than I did. Is it entitlement I wonder? Did her profession help make her a confident woman who was at home in the world? Again I felt like a newly arrived immigrant, awkward and unsure of how to position my body and my words.

"Connie," she said. "I'm glad to get away from the meetings for a while. Some of them are so dull. Let's find a quiet place to talk."

I noticed her impeccable outfit, jewelry and warm face. I hoped I didn't look as disheveled as I felt; I decided to keep my dark, unbuttoned raincoat on. "There's a coffee stand behind the escalators. Let's go there." We bought our coffee, found a secluded table and spent the first few minutes talking about our families. Nancy had two grown children, a boy and a girl. She also had a needy and distant mom who had recently gone into an expensive assisted living complex. Their relationship was stormy and Nancy was uncomfortable talking about her.

"How is your first book coming along? Any luck finding a publisher? I think it's so wonderful that you're writing. It's something I would love to do, too, if I had more free time."

"There was so much of Christine in that book." I clutched the bag on my lap that held a copy of the manuscript, uncertain if I wanted her to read it yet. "So, how do you think we could write about Christine?"

"Well it's really about us three women coming of age isn't it? Christine taught me so much about how to be the kind of physician I want to be – finding a human way to heal. She really was an amazing woman whom I grew to love."

"You have a unique side as her physician. It's a side I don't know about. What I know is how she affected me as her older sister. How I changed watching her die. How death no longer scares me the way it used to."

"It's Christine who became so strong in finding her voice. She called the shots, not the virus. I watched her become the decision maker. She told me what medications she wanted to try and which ones she didn't. She came up with her own health plan. She was determined to do things her way and I was her coach."

"How can we get the three sides of the story together? I don't know how it's going to work. Christine did leave a couple of journals I want to use. Should we write separately and put them together or should we write together by sharing pages via e-mail? Maybe we could get an exchange going. Let me get some paper out so I can take notes; I don't want us to forget anything." I pulled out my notepad and pen from my handbag and started writing. I was excited about working with another writer but I was also hesitant. Whose book would this really be?

"I think we should just write what we need to write separately. We won't know what that is until we write it. There's no way to control that now. I'm really overloaded at the university. Between my medical students and the clinic I don't want to give up I simply don't have the time I'd like to devote to this project. I can't do anything serious about this until next summer. I want to try and get all her medical records and go over them. There's so much there."

"I wouldn't know how to tackle that side of her story. Sometimes I cry just thinking about her nightstand full of pills. Jason was so funny this morning when I told him we might be writing a book together. He said, 'Mom, all right but don't smudge up the ink with tears going down your face!' I didn't know what to say."

"Jason knows how much Christine meant to you. Her story is one of hope – she spent all her time trying to get well. She lived as long as she did because of that hope and courage."

"I can't help but think of her as a victim sometimes even though I know she was courageous and all that. Her life was one hardship after another. Why did the virus strike her? You know when I asked her for a title she said, *Little Girl Lost*. Do you think she felt like a victim?"

"No, no, no I really don't. Once she saw what she had to deal with, she just took it over like it was one more thing to overcome. I think she thought she was going to beat this. She called the shots, not me or you or her family."

"But still I feel she had the cards stacked against her. Isn't that a terrible fate?"

"I don't know. All anyone can do is try and cope with what life brings –fairly or unfairly. Maybe Christine became a whole person because of her struggle with her disease. Maybe she began to heal from her painful past by moving towards a simpler life."

"She had to have the disease in order to become a whole person? I just can't buy that."

"That's the way it worked out. Her journey in finding her voice came through her illness. Would she have found it anyway? I don't know – I only know I would have never met her otherwise."

"I'd rather have her alive without a voice than dying with a voice." I said wondering how I would manage to write anything even as I was moving my pen across the white paper under my left hand. In large dark letters I wrote: "coming of age, three women, dying, self-discovery, voice, a good death."

"That's not your choice or my choice though is it?"

"I wanted her to grow old with me, that's all."

"We all want that."

"I guess you're right." I wondered if that's what our moms wanted too. How come they didn't get to grow old around the people they loved the most? Did our distant moms drive us so far away that there was no turning back? Was dying among strangers their fate all along? My heart reeled with the idea of fate and what could possibly be in store for me. My fingers moved away from my cup and settled onto the briefcase on my lap.

"I've brought a copy of my first book. Would you like to read it? There's no hurry in getting it back to me." I gently lifted the manuscript from my lap and put it on the table between us.

"It'd be an honor. I'll take it back with me; maybe I'll start it on the plane. I probably should be getting back to the workshops."

I picked the bound pages up off the table and placed them in her outstretched hands. For a moment we both stare at the cover, my mournful passport - photograph when I was twenty. I looked as miserable as I felt then, single and unexpectedly pregnant without future plans. My heart tugged as if I was offering a piece of it to her

"I'll take good care of it and get it back to you by the end of the year. I'm glad we got together. Everything will work out just fine." Nancy got up and pushed her chair in. We embraced good-bye with the manuscript between us.

I pick up the marbled drug journal once again and the irony of the word 'drug' hits me: Sal's illegal drug use gave her the virus yet it was drugs that kept her alive. In the end she was addicted to morphine and worried over this.

"I hate drugs. I don't want to take any of them. I hate the people who are hooked on them - what it does to them - and now here I am addicted myself."

"But you need them to stop the pain. They're legal. Your doctor gave them to you." I said, knowing what we both knew: It didn't matter that she was addicted. Her life had reached its end; it might as well end comfortably with drugs.

The words in her journal look foreign: AZT, T-Cells, CMV, parasites, portacath and protease inhibitors. It's a language Christine learned to decipher well. It's a language I could only take in small doses while she was alive.

May 1992: Dr. prescribed anti-depressant Amitriptoline- puts me to sleep –can't get up mornings.

Sept.12, 1992: Starting drug trial study at Yale – blind study – you don't know what you're really taking. Pro's – you'll be watched closely and it's free. Con's – long term side effects from ?? Drug?

Sept. 17th, 1992: Stopped taking all drugs – got really sick to my stomach. Let me "clean out" my system for a while.
Dec. 2, 1992 T cell count 350.

(There's a blank page before the next entry almost a year later.)
Nov. 1993: T cell dipped to 100 – maybe time to take something but WHAT? Decided on DD1.

Dec.4, 1993: started feeling sick, very tired and diarrhea – called Dr. and she said to stop taking drug to see if it stops.

Dec.21, 1993: Diarrhea stopped somewhat, not as much as before – still feel very very tired. Glad to stop DD1 – pain in the ass to take- tastes terrible!

My stomach does a flip as I imagine gagging on all those too large pills Christine hated. My heart jumps at the thought of all those long hospital stays. Why was it so important for her to remember? Certainly her journal shows how much she wanted to live.

I don't remember Christine ever screaming in anger or crying out in pain. I wonder if this is a sign of strength or of weakness. Is it strength to hold anger and excruciating pain deep inside your body? Or is it weakness not to scream bloody murder outside your body? I used to think it was a weakness but now I don't know. Maybe it's a kind of courage I haven't yet had to muster. A kind of courage only the dying need. Maybe writing this book is kind of like dying: both end in completion. Both require a suspension of the everyday self. Both evolve into vessels, which must float out to sea on their own.

Months after I met Nancy at the Hyatt, our plan to write this book together didn't look good. I was in the middle of the first draft but Nancy hadn't been able to get beyond some pages she wrote during vacation. Should I go ahead and wait for her to catch up? Should I go ahead and push her ahead too or go ahead by myself?

I thought I needed the doctor to help tell Christine's story, but what I really wanted was Nancy's knowledge to explain the medical struggle that was so much a part of my sister's life. I didn't want to have to figure that out for myself. I didn't want to do what I'm doing now, sitting alone with her drug journal. Initially I told myself it was too mechanical, too factual, too boring. But the opposite is true:

the entries are as alive with her illness as anything I've read or written about Christine.

*Feb. 17,1994: Officially diagnosed with AIDS because of infection, cryptosporidum, considered an opportunistic infection – **oh well, the good part** – I qualify for Social Security disability & for state medical care.*

"*Oh well the good part!*" Christine's practical side amazes me. Now, one doesn't need an opportunistic infection before being diagnosed with AIDS. But in the early 90's an HIV person wasn't considered to have AIDS until they had an opportunistic infection, an infection that wouldn't bother a healthy body but one which could easily kill an HIV person, something like pneumonia or the measles. Now it's the number of T-cells or CD4 cells that determines classification. (The T-cells are crucial to the functioning of the immune system and are the main cells the HIV virus attacks. A healthy body usually has from 500 to 1600 T-cells.) According to the literature most illnesses don't develop unless the counts are below 200. The most Christine ever had once she started to record them was 350 in 1992. By 1994 she was down to 65 and in 1997 she had only 20 T-cells left.

The bad part about waiting before being officially diagnosed with AIDS was that Christine and thousands of others had to get worse before they qualified for state aid, before they could receive the medical attention and medications they so desperately needed. The good part about waiting was that we could pretend she'd never make the transition to full blown AIDS – another term which was common ten years ago. "Full blown" always made me uncomfortable; I imagined a balloon filled with poisonous gases punctured by a needle, people scrambling away in a panic.

It's not panic I feel now while I continue to read, but rather a small ache in the pit of my stomach. How much pain could a then forty- three year old woman take?

May, 1994: Went to specialist (related to parasite infection). I have some sort of blockage in bile duct causing the pain in my stomach. Taking a drug called Diltiazem – used for people with high blood pressure – seems to relax the muscle and stops the stomach pain.

June 2, 1994: Intense pain in stomach all night – even pills did not help – called Dr. –said to go to emergency room.

(Days later)

No pain since last Thursday – Endoscopy procedure to be done today to unblock blockage in stomach.

July/August: Feeling pretty good – no more pain in stomach – just bloated and uncomfortable feeling there. Started taking garlic pills and blue green algae along with other meds. Feeling really good lately! No more pain or diarrhea!

Christine had made it to June of 1994 and despite the physical set backs she was ready to began another part of her life. That summer she'd come to visit us in Chicago, continued on to California and returned to us several weeks later. She'd lived with us for six months before returning home to Connecticut where the last part of her journey would unfold. It included a trip back out west for the both of us.

Just yesterday I decided to e-mail the doctor with my decision. It went something like this: "Nancy I think it's best if we take separate paths on this book- writing project. In waiting for your section I've come to realize I need to write on my own as Christine's sister. I think we have separate books in us; I need to go ahead with mine. Besides we're on different schedules, making working together difficult. I hope you will understand my position. Please write back."

I needn't have worried. Nancy wrote back within an hour.

"I truly understand how you feel and have no trouble with your writing the book you need to write... I encourage you to do the creative work that you have to do... I have learned a lot from both Christine and you, and also value our friendship."

At first I was relieved; thank God she understood! But just as quickly I was also disappointed that I no longer officially had a partner. I no longer had the imaginary cushion of another person, a medical professional to add legitimacy to this story. I was not doing what I'd told Christine we'd be doing, writing this book with her doctor. How would this affect my promise to her? How would it affect my writing from now on? Where would this unwritten book go?

I suddenly realized that I couldn't have imagined doing this book on my own, not then, not at the beginning when Christine was dying and then later when she'd died. It helped the book idea to have a partner, someone knowledgeable and supportive. Maybe the promise was really for me, a commitment that I would write this book. Maybe the pain evident in her journal was something that would bring some understanding of what she was battling with for so many years, something I couldn't possibly share with her. Just as suddenly I'm reminded of a phrase by the often bed-ridden writer, Flannery O'Connor: "In a sense sickness is a place more instructive than a long trip to Europe, and it's always a place where there's no company, where nobody can follow."

Maybe the unwritten book lies within the hearts of my sister, her doctor and myself. Untouched by words, our love travels freely among the oceans of the world just like my sister's ashes that floated briefly before disappearing from view.

Sea Sisters Tour

August 6ᵗʰ, 1994: Getting ready to go cross- country! Feeling <u>really great</u>!
August 8ᵗʰ 1994: Leaving for trip cross- country – feel great.

Christine wanted to live, to travel across country and settle in California. The summer of 1994 turned out to be full of hope for a future despite or maybe because of her AIDS diagnosis. For a while Christine didn't feel much pain and anything seemed possible.

I remember the stop in Chicago to visit us. Christine looked terrific, and so did her boyfriend Andy who had finally agreed to drive her cross- country. She had met this wonderfully large, sweet man, years earlier, and he had become devoted to her even after finding out about her virus. I wonder how many men would be as kind-hearted and as generous.

During the time I was working in the flower shop I met a really good friend, Andy: He was a kind, gentle soul. He has stood by me during this whole ordeal and has been very supportive and we became very close. We joked and laughed a lot. We liked each other's company. I could honestly say we were in love. Till this day he is still here for me with a warm smile and a big hug.

Both were sun tanned, smiling and healthy looking. There's a photo of that time that remains one of my favorites. In it Christine has light brown shoulder length wavy hair, warm eyes, red lipstick on smiling lips and long silver and turquoise earrings with feathers. She's wearing a dark sundress with large rose- petaled flowers. Andy has an attractive neatly trimmed mustache and beard, short dark hair and a gold hoop earring in his left ear. He's wearing a white muscle man t-shirt with his smile and has his right arm comfortably draped over Christine's back. There's a wistful quality in their gazes almost as if they weren't used to getting what they wanted.

I remember being happy and relieved to see them looking so well. Happy she was finally living her dream and relieved she was not too sick to go. Christine had packed her black Mazda with her belongings and made hotel living arrangements with a women's support group near Los Angeles. On the way out west she bought a set of dishes and stuffed the box in her already cramped car. "I don't know why I bought them. It's the last thing I needed, but they were such a nice shade of blue." The plan was that Andy was going to help her get settled and then fly back east. It didn't work out that way.

Living with AIDS. That was the only life she had now. She wanted it be in a warm climate by an ocean. Often times she'd said, "Connie, if you lived out west or down south I'd come live with you," or "it's the cold and dreariness I can't take. I need the water and the sun." I felt the same way myself.

I wanted my sister to live how and where she wanted. "Go, go if that's what you really want to do. Don't wait for your dreams to come to you." Of course I was also talking to myself. Didn't I have my dreams come true now that Michael and I had our two babies? Didn't I still long for more? Didn't I soothe myself by writing in journals but also longing to write like a real writer, to be published, to be acknowledged?

Do it now, do it now, do it now a voice inside my heart told my sister and me. I sit at the computer and still hear the voice saying, *Do it now*. The sudden temptation is to not do it now, to stop, to get up and do something else. I let the feeling pass and decide to write more; partly I don't want to let go of that hopeful summer when Christine looked so good.

My heart also wanted a comfortable death for her, a death with close friends, family and her beloved doctor nearby. Her move out to California, where she knew no one, reminded me of my father. Once he had admitted himself into the hospital, had surgery to remove cancer from his colon, then appeared back home days later without having told anyone of his whereabouts. Had he thought he might die and didn't want others around? Or couldn't he accept the family care he would have received? Maybe he couldn't stand to have anyone see him so vulnerable, so susceptible to pain and illness. Did Christine feel the same way? In 1994 no one knew when her death would occur. We only knew that no amount of medical intervention would save her life, and she probably knew that too. Then most people died rather quickly – much quicker than Christine. Now, people talk about living indefinitely with AIDS, as if it were a manageable disease. If she had gotten the virus just a few years later she'd probably be alive today. Then it scared me to think of her in a hotel room hurting alone, just like it scares me to think of dying alone.

Andy also imagined how scared and lonely she would be if he left her in that dirty noisy hotel room she had found. They argued and Andy won. A few days after they arrived in Los Angeles I got a call.

"Con, this is your crazy sister, I'm calling to ask a favor. Can I come stay with you for a while? Andy doesn't want to leave me here, and I don't want to go back to Connecticut."

"What happened? What about those women who were going to help you?" I was pissed that she'd given up on her dream so quickly and that Andy was not supporting her. How could a dream be gone in a matter of days, for Christ's sake?

"Andy's gotta get back to work and if he's going to drive me back to Chicago then we have to leave now. I keep telling him to take the plane and leave me here like we planned but he won't. He's afraid something bad will happen to me in this hotel. This is the best place the women I talked to could come up with; maybe I can talk with them again but Andy is too upset to listen to me."

"Of course you can stay with us. We'll work it out. Of course you can come." Now I had to deal with this? Where would we put her? What if she got really sick? After I got off the phone I talked with Michael and told him we needed to take my sister in. I explained that there was no one else in the world I would do this for but I wouldn't have my sister be without a home. Michael agreed; he has always liked Christine. I told Jason and Mika who were only five and three then. I don't recall what their reactions were, but I recall feeling they were too young to have a dying aunt. Jason was to start kindergarten and Mika pre-school at the public school across the street the next month. I was to start taking education classes to get my teaching certificate. Michael was to continue to support all of us with his work for the city.

Christine moved here in late August and stayed with us for six months. It was the first time we'd lived together in twenty-eight years. How would we manage? How would the children and Michael manage? I needn't have worried.

We settled my sister in the downstairs recreation room. I decorated the room with a comfortable futon, quilt, books and flowers. I wanted her to feel at home. I wanted her to feel a part of our family. We soon got into a routine and Christine fit in easily. Later Michael said he liked having her around; she was easy to get along with, didn't get in the way, and made wonderful beef stews, lentil soups, and spinach pies. The kids remember the nearby mall where she'd take them to Fluky's for hot dogs and then to KB Toys for treats. Christine surprised me with her ease at getting around the big city. She had her Mazda with her and drove herself to doctor's appointments. I remember taking her to several different AIDS support groups, but each of them flopped.

"I have nothing in common with these younger black and Spanish women. They're mostly addicts with children and I can't feel sorry for them, especially the ones who are still using. Some of them are living on the street and selling themselves. It's not me. I never did drugs; I never sold myself. I'm so glad I don't have young children to watch me die, that my girls are grown. The other place you took me to on Belmont Avenue was full of gay men. What am I gonna say? 'Hi guys, I got AIDS too'? Talking to strangers isn't going to do any good anyway."

There wasn't a group for white divorced middle-aged ethnic working class straight women who got AIDS from their partners. But I kept trying. The best I could do was take her to B-HIV, an agency in Evanston. We talked with a sympathetic counselor who several years later would suddenly lose her older sister to an untreated brain tumor. I liked this young smiling Anne and thought she might be able to get Christine to talk about her feelings. But Christine was no longer young and no longer smiling. Later I'd join a family members support group and I was surprised at the low turnout. Is the wealthy North shore location embarrassed that they, the privileged, are not immune to AIDS? Or do they have enough money to conceal their secrets?

In September of that year my book group went on our annual AIDS walk. I invited Christine not sure how she would feel. I invited her not sure how I would feel. Would she feel on display as one of the "sick people?" It was a hot but glorious morning along Lake Michigan in downtown Chicago. Thousands of people were gathered, many in groups from work or with friends, most looked healthy but some didn't look well enough to breathe let alone walk. I glanced at a skeletal woman in a wheelchair nearby and noticed her orange sweatpants and red shirt. I wondered why she wanted to draw further attention to herself. I turned away and hoped Christine hadn't seen her, a reminder of what was ahead.

"We don't have to walk the whole 10 kilometers and we don't have to walk fast," I said suddenly tempted to sit this one out.

"I'm all right. We're here; let's just get on with it," she said quietly.

I walked alongside and behind Christine but not ahead of her most of the time. It was a beautiful day on the lake, sunny and blue as the water and sky met up with the bright clouds. I walked and talked with the other women about the books we'd been reading. We'd just finished *Pigs in Heaven* by Barbara Kingsolver and I had adored the story about identity and belonging. Soon we'd be reading The Delaney Sisters, women in their 100's who'd written their memoir together, *Having Our Say*. Talking about books was like talking about people, it was something I could do for hours. Christine lagged behind, staring out into the lake. She didn't have much to say even when others tried to strike up a conversation.

Around the Shedd Aquarium we realized we weren't turning back, but walking further along to Meig's Field. I was worried it was too much and said to Christine, "Let's not walk all the way around; let's head back to Monroe Street. We don't have to go the full distance."

"We made it this far, we might as well finish it all the way," she said.

I looked at her tired face behind her sunglasses. My heart knew this would be the only time we'd do the walk together, so I slowed down my pace and walked alongside her.

The sole comment she made in her journal was:

Did an AIDS walk today- feel good- except for headache that started in the evening, got worse, throwing up, etc. migraine.

The following month she entered her only comment about her stay with us.

In Chicago, feel really good – lots to see and do.
Second visit to Illinois Masonic Hospital, had pap smear. T-cells 65. But I feel fine.

While we were together we went to see the movie, "Boys on the Side," starring Whoopi Goldberg, Drew Barrymore and Mary-Louise Parker. Did I really take her to the movies to watch Parker die of AIDS among her women friends? Did I think there was a lesson in this for us? Why did she put up with my need to connect our experience with others going through a similar one? Suddenly an image of us sitting at the Lincoln Village theatre appears. We're up close, maybe too close to death to learn anything. Christine was upset even before the movie begins,

"Connie, look, there's a rat running under the chairs! It's huge!"

I looked over but didn't see anything. I put my feet up anyway just like Christine had done. "That's disgusting. I come here a lot with the kids and I've never seen a rat before," I said embarrassed that it was Christine who'd seen this rodent and not someone else. Throughout the movie I was on the lookout but didn't see anything on the floor except for popcorn, candy boxes, and spilled pop. After the movie I wondered if I should tell the management about the rat, but I decided against it. There was nothing they can do anyway. Instead we headed straight to the car and I broke the silence with a question.

"Don't you think Drew's character looks and acts like Kerry? All that wild living, the baby, and then settling down with a cop! Maybe your youngest will come around to a happy ending too." I didn't dare say that I was of course the wild Whoopi character tending my sister, the dying sweet Mary-Louise.

"A little bit. I sure hope she finds someone to love and take care of her. I hope to God she doesn't have to go to jail for her wild ways like in the movie." Perhaps she didn't dare to say that she probably wouldn't be around long enough to find out. Nor did she say that she hoped her death could be as simple as an empty wheelchair in an empty apartment.

The other night I watched the movie again at home this time and alone. I watched it with an intensity I didn't have when Christine was still alive and sitting next to me. I kept trying to imagine what was going through her mind while she was watching. "I'm the dying Mary-Louise, look how I've deteriorated, how skinny, how ugly I've become. This is my future." I watched this time and let the women come together and part with tender love. I watched Whoopi head for her packed car and California, where Mary-Louise had wanted to settle but never made it. Drew and the baby and her cop stayed in the Arizona desert, a place Christine also loved. The three women became mind, body and spirit in my heart. During the credits the song, "You Got It" by Roy Orboson played and the words, *anything you want, you've got it* made me cry. Wasn't that what I'd tried to do for Christine? Had it been enough? I wrapped myself tightly in the green fleece blanket on the couch and rocked myself to sleep.

Suddenly now at the computer, I'm hungry. It's only one o'clock and I don't have to pick up the kids until three. I tap save, pull back the chair, and head for the kitchen. I take a pot from the shelf, fill it with water and turn on the stove. I'll have some vegetable pasta with cheese and butter. While the water's boiling I go downstairs to check on the dryer. Sonny runs from the pile of dirty clothes when he sees me. I don't like the cat lying on our clothes. I don't like him living in the downstairs room that once belonged to Christine. His sister is gone and so is mine.

Every once in a while I'll see Sonny lying on the dirt where Mooney's buried under the tree in our backyard and I'll wonder, Does he remember his sister? Is there a bond that death will never break? I feel bad that I don't like Sonny more, but the feeling leaves quickly. The clothes in the dryer are still damp so I turn the dial for another 30 minutes. Upstairs the water's at a boil. I stir in a half box of pasta, wait and wonder.

How do I condense a life onto pages that will never breathe? How do I make sense of a life and death that will never really make sense, not in the way I want it to make sense. Not in a-b-c or 1- 2 -3 order. Luckily my pasta is done and I can eat instead. I take my bowl and sit in the dining room. I light two votive candles by Christine's picture as if I'm feeding her too. I light a stick of the Japanese incense she so loved. Soon the woody smell mixes in with the heat of the pasta, cheese and butter. I eat fast, a habit cultivated as a child and can't seem to change. Our father was a super- fast eater. No one could beat him when he'd announce an eating race. That included sopping up your plate with bread and holding it up against your chest for the losers to see, a clean white plate. A plate that always pleased my father and put a smile on his face. A plate that irritated my mother: she was a slow eater and never won at anything.

I finish my pasta but am still hungry. I go back for seconds after dismissing the unwelcome reminder to wait; it takes twenty minutes to feel full. I want to feel full now and quickly finish up the pot, put my clean white bowl and fork in the sink and get back to work. By now it's 1:30 – I've got another ninety minutes.

Clock watching bothers me but I do it anyway. I have post it notes all over the house to remind me to live in the now, that the present is all there is. I believe this to be true. It's just that I have a hard time keeping to this belief. My thoughts race ahead as if to beat themselves at their own game, the game of time. Who's got more time? Who's got more stuff to fill into that time?

Limitless time, eternity, makes me feel lonely. I don't know why. Did Christine feel that way too? How could she not have felt lonely? Is that different from feeling alone? To be lonely is to feel isolated and not a part of something, to be alone is to feel apart, but not necessarily isolated. I like feeling alone but I don't like feeling lonely.

Right now I'm feeling lonely. Memories of the last time I took Christine to her apartment quietly appear. Her apartment across from the beach, where she grew to love her solitude, where she could go to the bathroom with the door open and moan loudly if she felt like it. This was weeks before her death, when she was already living at Hospice in Branford. It was the apartment her youngest daughter tried to live in the summer after her mother's death. The apartment I stayed in when I came to visit. It was the apartment where her white haired cat Shag still lived after she had gone to Hospice.

"Come on Christine, I'll help you up the steps. Shag is upstairs waiting to see you." I was nervous she might fall and break something –she was so frail.

"I don't know if I can make it – my legs hurt and my feet are swollen. How come we drove this way? You didn't tell me we were coming here." Christine said, as she made no move to get out of the car.

"I thought you'd like to see your things, your cat. Come on, let me help lift you out of the seat. Watch the belt." I unbuckled the belt and pulled it over her head and reached for her hands as I gently pulled her out of the seat, careful of her head. Now I wasn't sure why I'd driven her to her former home. I imagined her missing her things, missing her cat, missing her life.

We made the climb: one step and rest; one step and rest. Her apartment was on the second floor with a turn at the top of the stairs. We got to the door and Christine held onto the wall as I let us in with her keys that she no longer had any use for. We stepped into a room full of dark silence.

It was a small two- bedroom apartment with a walk-in kitchen attached to a living room. It was comfortable and warm, something my sister had always been able to do with her many apartments: Pier I wicker furniture, southwestern turquoise and sand art, large colorful pillows and healthy cactus on the window ledge. I guided Christine to the couch and walked towards the window to pull up the mini-blinds and open the front door for light and fresh air. It smelled like used kitty litter. Christine held her nose and said, "Nobody's changed the box. I always cleaned it out once or twice a day."

"It didn't smell bad this morning. Let me do it now."

I put the clumps of litter in a plastic grocery bag out on the porch to take to the dumpster later. Everything in the apartment felt miniature size except for us. I peeked into the larger of the bedrooms, the one that used to be Christine's. Nothing had been moved, almost as if to say, "Your apartment's waiting for you to come back to when you get well" – or was it – "Your apartment won't be touched until you're gone." I wanted Christine to think the first, that her apartment would always be waiting for her, that she would regain her health and return, but I knew she wouldn't live there again. Of course she knew it too. Only we didn't ever speak of it out loud.

The bedroom was taken up by the queen- sized futon, which was covered by a white embroidered spread I'd given her. Many pillows were fluffed up and arranged neatly against the wall. The phone, lamp, loud ticking clock, books, magazines and no- longer- needed medicines were on a low nightstand. At the foot of the bed sat a wicker trunk full of pretty sheets and blankets. (She was always cold no matter how many blankets she had wrapped around her thin body.) Around the room were piles of clothing and baskets neatly filled with stuff. Directly across from the bed hung the painting I now wish I owned. It once belonged to our grandmother, Crysoula, for whom Christine was named, and eventually came to hang on my mother's wall until Christine asked for it. Had our Yiayia owned it when her handsome young husband, Anastas, died of influenza? Had it made the long train journey from California to his mother's house in Massachusetts? The ornate gold leaf frame held a painting of a blond white robed angel guarding a sweet red cloaked girl from the evil wolf in the woods. It was beautifully painted in deep maroons and browns and had a pleasing, mystical feel to it, as if it could protect the walls of its owner. I no longer know where the painting hangs. My youngest niece took it with her, but I don't think the white robed angel has been able to protect her.

The door to the smaller bedroom was closed. It was the room with the mattress on the floor where I used to sleep and where her youngest daughter and grandson sometimes slept in. It was filled with stuffed animals, toys and lost dreams.

I didn't see the cat anywhere.

"Shag, Shag, come here – Christine's here – come out." I said a bit too loudly.

"He's probably hiding under the bed. Just leave him alone. Here, help me get up to the toilet. I gotta pee bad."

I held onto both her elbows and led her to the bathroom, which was only steps away. I carefully positioned her bottom on the seat and closed the door to that tiny bathroom which had witnessed so much suffering over the past several years – nausea, vomiting, diarrhea, aches and pains of every body part imaginable.

"Shag! Come out, Shag!" I'm anxious to get this damn cat out of hiding. What was keeping it from running up to its owner of many years? Didn't he hear her voice? Sense her presence? I walked into the bedroom and peaked under the futon. At first I didn't see anything. I bent down on all fours and looked deeper. Ah, there he was, hiding in a corner. I reached in and took him out by the neck.

"Christine, here he is – I've got him! Look, look here!" Just as I was bringing him closer he wiggled out of my hands and ran back to the bedroom without a glance at his owner. I looked over at Christine who was walking on her own back to her chair by the window.

"Maybe he doesn't recognize me after all these weeks; maybe he's scared. I want to go now. It's not my place anymore; let's just go," she said as she tried to get up by herself.

My heart sank at this latest failure in my reunion plans. I longed to see Christine stroking Shag's long white hair and listening to him purr. I wanted to see a smile on my sister's face but I didn't think digging him out a second time would do any good. I looked over at the couch and startled myself. For a moment I'd forgotten, forgotten what my sister looked like.

Christine leaned back into the couch and closed her eyes. I stared at her features. Her nose- she'd always thought too large- was now indeed way too big. Her lips were small and pale. Her eyelids were huge and deeply carved into their sockets. Her chin was a sharp edged triangle. Her face was a sunken mess. She looked dead. Standing in her living room all I could do was stare, stare and wonder what kept her alive way past the point of enjoyment.

I also wondered what had happened to Shag. Was the smell of a decaying body already evident to him? Or had he simply let go of her? Did cats have memories?

Suddenly as I'm typing I remember another cat from my childhood. An outdoor cat my sister and I shared. My parents wouldn't have any animals inside the house. In many parts of Europe pets lived outside. *Treeha, treeha* or "hairs, hairs" my mom would say in Greek - always afraid of hairs getting on our food, hands or face. The cat's name was Peepena – a Greek name my mom had suggested – something about her having a cat in Greece with that name. Peepena was mostly black with white patches. One day Peepena got hurt – I don't remember how but I remember her lying in the front yard bleeding.

We ran inside, calling, "Mom, Peepena's hurt – we gotta do something!"

"Leave her alone and come inside," she said in Greek.

"But she's hurt – she needs help," I said.

"I don't want more trouble. She's a cat; she belongs outside. Leave her."

"But Mom, she's bleeding!" Christine said.

"Leave her. *Affesata. Then thelou fasareea.* Leave her; I don't want trouble," she said again in Greek. Her fear of trouble from my father was greater than her fear of life and death.

I don't remember what happened next. I only remember not seeing Peepena again. Years later when I was in high school my younger brother Tas had an outside dog who got run over by a car in front of our house. My mom again voted to avoid trouble and do nothing. But this time I was older and I had money from my library job. I called my friend and she came to pick up the bleeding dog that would leave permanent blood spots on her upholstery. My brother was ten and in love with his dog. We got in the car too, but I don't remember what happened. I only remember the dog lived.

Christine lived another four years after her return to Connecticut in 1995. After months with us she was homesick for her children, her grandchild, her boyfriend, her things. That year there was new hope for a cure: pro-tease inhibitors were introduced and soon infected patients were living longer but it was several years too late for Christine. Her virus was too advanced. She began taking them anyway with mixed results.

Our Sea Sisters Tour took place in April of that year, the one time we were in California together. It was a trip I didn't want to take at the time. My life felt chaotic staying at home with my children, searching for work and wondering what had happened to my marriage. Michael and I had become mom and dad and there was no room for anything else. It was a role that suited Michael, but not me. I needed more. Writing seemed like part of that more but it felt like a dream. Meanwhile Christine's dream of traveling down the coast tugged at my heart as if to say, "Take her to see what she wants to see. You'll regret it if you don't. Do this for her now. There's no one else who'll take her."

California was the place my grandparents loved, the land where my mother's three siblings were born and the land we might have called home had not my grandfather died, leaving my mother without a father. Recently my cousin had been talking about unclaimed territory around Los Angeles that once belonged to our grandfather's family, land that should have been a part of our mother's legacy, the land my sister ached to live and die in.

How was anyone to know that both my grandfather and sister would take similar journeys across the continent to die of catastrophic plagues? Was it merciful to have our grandfather die a quick death of influenza and less merciful to have my sister die a slow death from AIDS? In 1918 there wasn't much that could be done for the infected; one either survived it or died like millions around the world did.

Gina Kolata who wrote about influenza in the book *FLU* says, "The epidemic puts every other epidemic of this century to shame. It was a plague so deadly that if a similar virus were to strike today, it would kill more people in a single year than heart disease, cancers, strokes, chronic pulmonary disease, AIDS and Alzheimer's combined. It killed more Americans in a single year than died in battle in World War I, World War II, the Korean War and the Vietnam War." And yet, she goes on to say, the epidemic remains a hidden part of our history, almost as if the world wanted to forget the tragedy. I wonder if AIDS will be treated in a similar way years from now. I wonder if my sister will merely be a number, part of the twenty-five million who have already died worldwide from this latest plague.

And so we flew into Sacramento where my friend Bram had agreed to drive us down the coast along Highway One. He lived there in a beautiful old home with his long-time companion Kermit. It was big favor to ask of him, but one he readily agreed to, even after his recently discovered heart problems. (Our then almost thirty year friendship was firmly cemented in journeys by car. In the 70's we'd driven several times to California and New York, and in the 80's we'd driven through Sweden, Germany, France and Italy. Bram drove, I rode.)

In California my girlfriend Janice flew down from Seattle to be with us before we began our drive down the coast. I remember the ache I felt for my family of friends.

They'd helped make this trip seem like a normal vacation instead of a dying sister's last wish. The weight of the wish was heavy on my heart. We woke up early one morning when everyone else was still asleep, made coffee and settled into the sunlit living room heavy with comfortable sofa chairs, leather couch, books, bright flowers, and original pieces of art from around the world. It was a room I could easily have lived in. Janice looked wonderful in a flowing African print robe. Six months apart to the day, we'd been friends since we met as waitresses the summer of 1972 when we were twenty- four with long hair, long dreams and short skirts. I felt older and heavier now in layers of clothing. We were facing each other on the couch by the window. My legs were crossed and under me. Janice's were turned towards me with her knees on the couch. We began to talk like my sleeping sister and I never could.

"Do you think she's preparing to die?"

"I don't know. If it were me, I'd be freaking out. She's so quiet it's kind of scary. I don't know if she's terrified or if the drugs she's taking have dulled her senses." I said.

"What will it be like when we die? I can't imagine. Fifty is the beginning of middle age, and I still have both my parents alive, haven't had to go through what you did with your father."

"I never imagined death this way- part of everyday life. As if it's as natural as breathing. My father fought the whole way, so it seemed like death should be a battle to the end. He was like a shoeless soldier fighting off the booted monster." I said. I realized death was a part of everyday life no matter how it was dealt with, but I didn't want to give more power to death than it already had in scaring me out of my wits.

"Maybe when we're in our sixties we can begin to imagine our own deaths. It won't seem so foreign. Maybe we'll have gotten used to the idea that one day we'd simply cease to exist." Janice said.

"I wish I believed in a heaven; it would be reassuring," I said, knowing there was no heaven with angels and white clouds awaiting any of us.

"Does Christine believe in an afterlife? Is she spiritual?"

"She says she is sometimes. I'm afraid we've adopted my father's beliefs instead of my mother's. He went to church in case there was a God; and she went because she knew there was. I don't know why doubt wins over certainty in so many battles, maybe because doubts create the desire to search for answers. Certainty is the opposite, there's no need for answers."

"That's why religion and spiritual things can't be discussed rationally or intelligently. Faith is not something that can be understood with the mind," Janice said.

"Unity has taught me not to be afraid of uncertainty, that it's all right to live with the unanswered questions and what we say to ourselves is what really happens, the "our thoughts are prayers" kind of thing. So with all my questions and doubts what does that make me?"

"A skeptic like your father!" Janice said with a hearty laugh. She got up to refill our cups and suddenly I was aware of the large pottery platter on the coffee table in front of me. It was filled with many paperweights of different shapes and colors. Sunlight streamed in and the yellows, oranges, blues and reds within each glass sphere glistened and danced around the sand- toned platter. I watched and thought there was no more beautiful thing on earth.

The next morning we said good-bye to Kermit and Janice. Christine and I settled into Bram's bright red Saab and we began our trip down the coast. I sat in the passenger seat and Christine settled in the back seat with pillows, blankets, Kleenex, garbage bags, water bottles and her large sack of medicines. She didn't complain and seemed happy to have us navigate, leaving her to stare out the window and live inside her dream. I was fearful that we'd have to take my sister to the emergency room or that Bram might not be up to the long drive. I needn't have worried. Despite Christine's

86

stomach cramps and weakness she loved being in the abundant sunlight. That's what Bram remembered most about our trip, lots of sun, Christine's pleasure and his desire to travel to just about anywhere. When we arrived in San Francisco I was anxious to point out the sights.

"Wake up, Christine, we're on the Golden Gate Bridge. Look, here's Fishermen's Wharf. Remember the "flowers in your hair" song we used to love? We're here!"

Christine didn't say much but I knew by how she was looking that she was taking it all in. Soon she said, "I've got an address of an AIDS clinic here I'd like to check out to see if they have any new information."

Bram quickly said, "We can do that. Just give me the address."

I was reluctant to go, fearful Christine might have resurrected her plan to live in San Francisco. What if someone said, "Sure come stay with us, we'll find a cheap place for you to live in by the ocean and we'll put you on these new protease inhibitors that will keep you alive longer."

We found the clinic under an expressway and walked up the dark stairs to the office. Christine asked if someone was available and soon a woman came out and took her into a back office. An hour later she came out with her head down carrying a bunch of papers. She looked too tired to make it down the stairs. How could she possibly think of living alone here where she knew no one?

"Well, there's some new stuff out, but it's only in trials. As far as living here, it's impossible without a lot of money." She sat down next to us and our eyes locked for a moment before she continued, "I'll ask Dr. Angoff about this new medicine when I get back. Let's keep driving around I want to see everything," she said.

She tapped me on the shoulder and said quietly, "I wish I'd come earlier; I wish I could start over again."

"We should've both come in the 70's," I said imagining another kind of life that included a healthy sister owning a hip flower shop in Haight Ashbury. Maybe even a women's bookstore for me.

We got back in the car and drove down Castro Street, the famous gay community, and Bram told us about some of the wild parades he'd attended. We stopped at City Lights Bookstore where Ferlingetti and so many other poets and writers of the '60's had hung out. We ate in a cute Italian place with delicious pasta, but Christine only picked at her food.

In San Francisco we spent two nights with Jay and Brian, friends I'd made at the same restaurant I'd met Janice in all those years ago. As soon as we arrived Christine wanted to go in the backyard to lie in the sun and relax. She wasn't much on talking and I hadn't seen these friends for years. Bram knew them also, so we sat down to wine and conversation. They knew my sister was sick but they didn't know what was wrong with her.

Brian - still handsome- was the one to ask.

"AIDS," I said. "She got it from an old boyfriend with a drug habit. He's dead." I sounded as if I were talking about someone I wasn't related to.

"That's terrible. Is she OK now? What can we do to help her out?" Jay said. She was still gorgeous, her hair still long and wavy, her eyes bright and a warm smile.

I didn't say anything for a moment. I stared at this handsome couple who'd been together for almost twenty years. They seemed so much in love still, the looks, the gentleness and the concern they expressed towards each other. Suddenly I wondered if never marrying made a couple work harder at keeping the relationship alive and growing. Marriage seemed to stifle growth and I didn't know how to keep mine alive and breathing. I was relieved to be away from the stress of couplehood but I missed my young children. I wasn't sure how to respond.

"Not right now. She needs lots of rest and room to spread out. Don't take it personally if she doesn't keep the conversation going," I said.

"Just let us know if there's anything we can do." Brian says.

"She'll tell us if she needs anything. She's pretty good at that," Bram said.

"Mostly she wants to tag along and not have to decide anything." I said. Suddenly I remember her voice so often pleading with me, "Mom says I can go with you, please let me come too." My forehead would wrinkle and I'd say, "No, I don't want you with me, stay home. Get away." Now I wonder if a big sister would have done the same to me.

Days later we were on the road again, traveling towards Santa Cruz, Monterey, Morro Bay, Santa Barbara, Malibu: beautiful coastal towns with fancy shops, museums and gardens. The views were magnificent and Bram and I took many pictures. Christine was enjoying herself. Was a part of her disbelieving that she was really in her dream, that she was really in California traveling down route 1?

It was in one of these towns that I picked up the plastic sea mermaids for Mika. One was turquoise with brown hair and the other pink with blond hair. They were linked together and the sticker behind them read, *Sea Sisters.* (I don't recall what else it might have said since they disappeared into the give-away box years ago.) Christine and I laughed at these silly plastic maidens and when we told Bram he said, "Hey those mermaids could easily be you two, the two water-loving sisters. Let's call this trip, "The Sea Sisters Tour!" And from then on that's how we referred to our Pacific coast adventure.

It was also along the way to San Diego that we stopped to take the photo of us in the Pacific Ocean. We were in the town of Carmel with rainbow flags flying outside expensive boutiques. We stopped to put our feet in the ocean and Bram snapped the *Sea Sisters Forever* photograph.

I have the pewter framed photo to my left on the table while I'm writing. I like looking at it – the vastness of the ocean, the smiles on our sun-glassed faces, and the large dark boulder behind us. We're positioned the same way we were over thirty years ago on the east coast when we were still children and I towered over my little sister. The distance between us in the grown up photo is so much less. Our t-shirts are almost touching; our shoulders do touch. In three decades we have managed to become about as close as we could become. We grew up together, but apart. Different paths, different endings, but always sisters.

Looking at the photograph I see the vastness of the ocean that takes up most of the frame. I see the large waves forever caught in mid-air. Those waves were meant to crash down onto the shore and disappear. Maybe they're not unlike us humans pretending to be large waves that will last forever. Did we forget we were meant to crash onto the earth and become one with it? Did we once know this to be true? Suddenly I remember a phrase I'd re-discovered recently from a forgotten source.

I once thought that when you understood something, it was with you forever. I now know that isn't so, that most truths are inherently unattainable, that we have to work hard all our lives to remember the most basic things.

Must we work hard all our lives to remember that death is not our enemy? That life is a part of death? That most truths are elusive and only arrive when we are ready to hear them over and over again?

Christine's life and death taught me about impermanence. Before her death I walked around believing that I would somehow live forever, not unlike believing that if we just lived right nothing terrible would happen to us. There were plenty of people who lived right and had terrible things happen to them: sudden deaths, accidents, diseases, madness. I had no powers to keep her alive. I had no powers to keep terrible things from happening. I only had the power to make her more comfortable: going on doctor's appointments, taking her places, sending flannel nightgowns, flowers, People magazines. In making her comfortable I also made myself more comfortable with the idea of my own death, not unlike the wave in the photograph which of course did crash into the ocean and my sister who years later did become a part of two oceans.

Our trip was a success. We sunned ourselves on the beach in Santa Barbara, just as we had done countless Sundays at the beach on Long Island Sound. Between the sun and sand, my sister and I were soothed into a cocoon of warmth that remains until this day. We didn't see everything and we didn't do everything, but we were happy to travel as passengers on the coastal highway. One disappointment was in San Diego where they say the sun always shines. On the day we were there it was raining.

Baptism by Fire

It was hard work caring for three babies at such a young age. I was a baby myself! It was very hard for me to cope with caring for them and with Theo's (gambling) problem. At times I would get so angry! I didn't know how to be a mother! My parents were no help. They were the last people I wanted to be like.

Yet looking back now, I see I had my father's hot temper and my mother's patience at times. I shut up and did what I was told as she did.

She would always hope and pray my father would change and I also thought the same about Theo. "Never give up," she would say.

One Saturday in October my eighty-two year old friend and I go to hear Studs Terkel, who had just written a book on death and dying, *Will the Circle Be Unbroken?* When I invited her she said, "Oh I knew Studs way back in the 50's on the south side. We were all in the civil rights movement together." I picked up my friend, who was also named Christine. Walking into Unity we bumped into the famous, white haired author.

"Studs, remember me? Christine? We sat on the bus together several years ago and we were in the newspapers together." She rushed over to embrace him and at first he stared at her but then his eyes widened and he said, "Of course! How the hell are you?" He opened his arms to walk into her embrace, and I was delighted to watch the excitement of people decades older than myself. I wanted to grow older with that excitement still intact.

Christine was smiling her wide smile and she looked radiant. Each time I looked at her I was amazed at her oh-so- smooth skin on her face and hands. She and Lena Horne could have been sisters. I only wish I would age as gracefully, but years of sun bathing had left my skin wrinkled with age spots. I suddenly flashed on my sister and wished she, too, had the opportunity to age, gracefully or not.

We walked up to the sanctuary and the place was packed. Christine led and I followed her to her usual spot to the left of the pulpit. We sat and I showed her the book.

"This is so exciting. I just love being here with all these intelligent people."

For me, just watching Studs smile, talk with Reverend Ed and remember all that he remembered was entertainment enough. I had a hard time imagining myself as alert at his age. He began by telling a joke.

"Two people are talking and one asks, 'Heck who'd want to live to be ninety? That's so old.' Studs chuckles and says, "Everyone whose eighty-nine that's who!"

Christine took my arm and said, "That's so true. We all want to keep on living; I'm going to make it to one hundred!"

I squeezed her arm and silently prayed that she would succeed, even though my sister hadn't. My thoughts traveled to a time when my sister was still alive.

We were in her cozy apartment on the beach, watching an old home movie of our parent's wedding and Christine's baptism. The black and white movie was originally an old reel I had converted into a video. It began, with fast, out- of- focus images of the bride and groom. Light flashed off of my mom's gold fillings and her face was full of smiles. Her long satin gown complimented my dad's tuxedo. Quickly they disappeared, and Christine appeared at her party. She was the center of attention as the curly headed beauty. She's not a baby but a toddler. (It wasn't until later that I discovered her baptism certificate and realized she had been sixteen months old, an unusual occurrence in the Orthodox church since baptisms are generally done in the first six months to protect the baby's soul. Did my parents fight over her name, and which church she'd be baptized in, like they had with my younger brother?) Christine was quiet watching herself. I made comments like, "How beautiful you were; everything is beautiful about you!" She smiled and wanted to watch it again. There was a sadness in her eyes as if to say, It's all gone, all those years in between are gone, gone just like I will be gone soon, too. This sudden truth keeps me from inspecting her too closely. Instead I imagined the feelings that might have been in that curly-headed beauty's heart. Young Christine's thoughts might have gone something like this:

I remember cold air against my skin as my clothes were being removed. The ceremony was long, wet and greasy. The incense hurt my nose. The body dunks into the golden basin of water was scary and the olive oil swabs all over my body tickled. I'm wrapped in a large new white towel. My godparents Clara and Pete dressed me in a white crinoline dress with ruffles. Then they put a large gold cross around my neck. The metal was cold but maybe my soul had just been saved from the fires I would someday face.

I remember the party and how everyone wanted a turn holding me. My head was full of curls and I looked like a kewpie doll. I was afraid to go to my father's mother. I started to cry as I was being handed to Maya. She was very thin and wore only black. She had no teeth and her lips were inside her mouth. I cried some more and then was handed to my other Grandma, my Yiayia whom I liked. She was plump and wore a holiday dress in bright colors. She wore jewelry that sparkled. I was supposed to be named after her, Crysoula; it means gold in Greek. I don't know how I wound up with Dorothy Christine. Yiayia had big ears and large hands to hold me with. It was a party to honor me. It was the only time I remember being the center of attention. I don't know why my mother wasn't holding me.

My heart aches while imagining what my baby sister might have felt. Early in her journal she talks about our mother's lack of warmth.

My mother seemed to virtually ignore my feelings. Her thinking was to put on a happy face (no matter what), dress up nice, go to church, and everything would be all right. I guess the only way she knew was how she had been brought up. My grandmother was the same. Nevertheless, she (my mother) did the best she could, under the circumstances.

I remember my mother fussing with my hair every morning. I had naturally curly hair, yet she would make pipe curls. I hated them! She would not let me cut my hair. I think I was about thirteen when she finally agreed to let me cut it.

Christine's long curly hair was something I envied as a child. Especially since all the grown ups would crowd around to touch her beautiful crown of curls. My brother Jim had curly hair too and hated it. Tas and I had straight hair. My mother would spend hours tying up my hair in long white strips of old sheets so I would have pipe curls for church. It never worked for long. One time when I was about ten I had my first Tonette permanent and I was a head of silly curls. My father went nuts and yelled at my mom for paying good money to make me look bad.

In a letter Christine's friend Margie remembers her long hair too.

I remember when our first fight started. It was over the guy who lived down the street. His name was Dominick Robles. Both Christine and I liked him; then we found out he liked Christine because of her beautiful long hair. I had short hair. Oh I remember telling her one day when we were mad at each other that I was going to come to her house and cut her hair, so she went in the house and came out with a pair of scissors and said, "Go ahead, but my father will kill you!" We looked at each other and started laughing.

Now, sitting at Unity with another Christine who also had only daughters, I wonder: did the child in white feel protected with the golden cross around her neck? Did the child fear for her life? Did the child feel loved? The gold may have been too heavy; the fear may have become the dark Grandma forecasting doom; the love may have passed on from one hand to another, leaving my sister unprotected, fearful and unloved.

She must have felt she had been thrown to the wolves when she was married at fifteen, went to bed with a stranger, when her parents gave up on raising her. Instead of being a high school student worried about passing her history test or finishing a book report, Christine was forced to struggle with grown-up problems.

Many times I tried to save money. We moved around a lot and I thought having my own home would make things O.K. Theo would always take the money I tried to put away, he would say it was his. Things got out of control. We were even evicted once for not paying the rent (he told me he was paying it.)

One day he gave me a lot of money and told me no matter what, don't give it to him. Then when he came storming in one night demanding the money, I said "No," and got knocked around. I was pregnant. (I gave him the money.) From then on I didn't want his dirty stinking gambling money. I wanted to flush it all down the toilet!

By then I thought I had had enough. I wanted to leave him, but where would I go? There were no places for women to go like today. I certainly didn't want to go back home—never!

I gave birth to my third daughter Kerry when I was twenty. March 26,1972. Theo wasn't there when I gave birth – didn't know where he was – he was kind of disappointed it wasn't a boy. Besides, he thought being in the delivery room was disgusting.

I was so proud! I loved having three daughters! I never really wanted a son. My girls were so beautiful when they were born.

Theo didn't want me to take birth control pills. He said it would poison my body, but after the third one I started taking them secretly. He would have me pregnant till he had his son! No thanks!

When Kerry was about a year old, we took a trip to visit my in-laws in Greece. My mother and brother Jim came also. Theo stayed home and worked.

My in-laws were warm, loving people and Greece was so beautiful! Kerry was baptized in an old Greek Church; Theo's sister Maryann was the Godmother.

My father paid for the trip.

As the years passed there were good and bad times.

We finally got the house I wanted – with a pool – the girls were really happy.

It was far away from Bridgeport and my parents. (Not as far as I wanted, but it would have to do for now.)

Gambling was still a problem. Theo finally admitted he couldn't control it, and needed to be away from the people who gambled.

After two years we sold our home and made plans to move to Florida. Theo wanted to work down there, but then found out you can't really make money at his trade the way you can in Connecticut. He was really a good chef at this point. He never went to school for it but he learned by doing and caught on fast.

We went to Florida for a week, looked at houses, jobs etc. The girls loved it and I loved the climate.

He decided for me and the girls to move down there and he would stay in Connecticut and work and send money. (Looking back now that sounds good, but back then I was terrified of being alone without him!) Anyway what would that solve? How could I trust him? He would surely start to gamble again. What would I do if the money didn't come?

Throughout the years Theo borrowed lots of money from my father. He said it was a loan but he never paid him back. I guess he thought my father "owed" it to him. That really didn't bother me at the time, "that serves my father right," I thought, he wanted me (forced me) to marry this man. "Good," I thought. (Bit of vengeance there!)

My life was in utter turmoil. What to do? Move to Florida without him? We sold our house to the very first buyer, so we had to move. I started to panic. So much I did not know about this strange place Florida. How would I manage alone? After many weeks of thinking I decided to stay in Connecticut. (At least I was familiar with it.)

Thinking back now - _What Was Wrong with me_? This was my _chance to leave_! Somehow I just couldn't do it alone.

Leaving now would be almost impossible. Theo would always put me down (like my father often did.)

"Who would want a woman with three kids? You don't even work. You can't do anything to support yourself."

He was right. My self- esteem was really low; I was beginning to think I couldn't do anything right. My father and Theo were right. I was a stupid nobody.

We found a rental apartment in a quaint town called Branford. The schools were good and the girls loved it there. We lived near the center of town and could walk there. I liked it too.

Throughout the years Theo would always criticize this country; he said it ruined him. He always talked about going back to Greece. That was the life, not America.

I didn't like when he said things like that. Life is what you make it, I thought, no matter where you live, America or Greece.

After a few years of living in Branford Theo had a plan to move to Greece and open a tourist restaurant on the island of Mykonos. He would leave us here and said he would send money. Oh no, I thought, not again!

I didn't want him to leave, but that didn't matter to him. He promised he would send for us when the time came.

I remember pleading, begging him the night before he was to leave. Don't go! I can't do this alone! Please! But his mind was made up; he was leaving.

That was the last straw!!

He left some money for us to live on, but after awhile the money was gone. Theo told me that my father would give me money and he would pay him back. HA!

I hated the thought of asking my father for money and didn't till I was really desperate. My father gave me a hard time about it. Again I thought, 'Hey, you wanted me to marry this guy.'

I decided I wasn't going to beg for money anymore, I was too proud for that and I didn't believe in welfare.

Through neighbors I found a job selling flowers outside, in front of Yale New Haven Hospital. There were long hours on hot sunny days – sometimes 9 –10 hours a day – but I loved it. I was making my own money! Finally, I thought to myself, I'm worth something!

I started to come alive! People thought I was smart and pretty- <u>me</u>!

I was my own person- not Theo's wife, I was "Christine." I started feeling attractive and looking "good." I even started going out with friends.

Somehow I couldn't think of going back to my old lifestyle. For once in my life I was really happy!

It was at this time I decided to get a divorce. I could do it, I thought. I could make it on my own!

This was soon after I'd married Michael, around 1980. I remember the conversations we'd have on the phone. I didn't want Christine to feel she had to stay married for the sake of her children and neither did she. That was what our mom had done and we both vowed not to repeat her mistake. Or at least what we thought was a mistake at the time. I remember saying, "Christine do what you feel is best for you, what your heart tells you to do. The girls will be all right. Just do what you gotta do. Come to Chicago and we'll help you out."

My sister Connie wanted me to move to Chicago with the girls, I thought about it and decided against it. How I wish to God I had left then. My whole life would have gone in a different direction and I probably would not be sitting here at 4 o'clock in the morning frantically writing all this down. I don't think I have too much longer, and I wanted my daughters to know the truth about my life – You see, I have AIDS.

On May 26 1981 the divorce decree was final. I know this because I'm looking at the torn three-page judgment in front of me. The print is typed on a manual typewriter. The marriage lasted thirteen years, longer than I had anticipated. Christine was twenty-nine years old.

The divorce decree came when my nieces were twelve, eleven and nine, difficult years; the same ages my son and daughter are now. God, how they would hurt if they were suddenly separated from their father. Did my nieces feel the same way? Did my nieces ever forgive their mother? The oldest never did. She carried the hurt and carries it still. The youngest was wounded long before the divorce. The middle one Tina remains the healthiest and happiest – her mom's golden girl.

I look down into the yellow folder I've marked "Christine's original documents" and see I also possess her birth and marriage certificates, passport, immunization record, high school equivalency diploma, certificates in advanced floral design and her death certificate. Also two perfect attendance awards from when she was 12 and 13. She was proud of those.

Does a life get reduced to the papers that are left behind? If she had more diplomas and certificates would her life have meant more? I don't know. I only know this folder doesn't hold all that my sister meant to me.

Isn't that why Christine decided to write h. journal on the night she thought she'd die? Isn't that why both adore and detest the act of writing? I adore thinking about writing, I adore reading what others have written, and I adore the idea of writing. What I sometimes detest is the actual lonely work of writing. I suppose it's not unlike the loneliness of dying. The long hours of sitting, the long hours of waiting, not knowing when inspiration or a peaceful end will arrive. That writing night in March of 1998, Christine must have felt that way too.

I'm forty-six years old, yet I feel that I've lived a whole lifetime and sometimes more. I have been through so much, starting at a very early age, so much pain, so much suffering. Why? I'm tired. Enough is enough. I don't want to suffer anymore. I don't want to struggle anymore.

Isn't that why Mitch Albom wanted to see his old professor, before he left for good? In the popular memoir, *Tuesdays with Morrie*, Mitch re-established their long- ago friendship as the former teacher answered questions about life.

"But can I tell you the thing I'm learning most with this disease? [He had Lou Gehrig's disease.] The most important thing in life is to learn how to give out love, and to let it come in. Let it come in. We think we don't deserve love, we think if we let it in we'll become too soft."

Let love come in. It sounds so simple.

Maybe that's what I'm doing now writing about Christine, allowing our love to flow without barriers between us.

Later on in the book Morrie says, "The truth is once you learn how to die, you learn how to live." Learning how to die is not something I'd ever thought about. The idea intrigued me. I wondered if I could ask my dying sister similar life and death questions.

How does it feel to be dying? Morrie was an old man in his late seventies. Christine was thirty years younger. He'd had three more decades to live and get used to the idea of death. Do you ever get used to the idea of your own death?

How would the big sister – little sister dialogue go? I'm going to live and you're not, how do you feel about that? What would I want her to say? I suppose I wanted her to put into words her anger or resolve or whatever else she was feeling. I needed words to make sense of the nonsensical. But I suppose the question really was: Did Christine need words like I needed them? Or was she wise enough to know nothing with or without words would ever make sense again?

Nothing made sense when I talked with my mother one morning before Christine's death, soon after I had told her Christine wanted to be cremated. It was five a.m. Eastern Standard Time. I jumped up and caught the phone on the third ring.

Kale Mera, she shouted in Greek. Long distance calls made my mother shout, regardless how good the connection was. When she called her aunt in Greece we had to leave the room it was so loud.

"Good morning to you too, Mom. What's up?"

"Don't let her burn the body. Don't burn the body. It's a sin and she can't do it!"

"What are you talking about?" I knew what she was saying but I didn't want to make it easy for her. Doing the right religious thing came before the wishes of her daughter. (Later when I asked the priest again why cremation was frowned upon he said it's because Jesus wasn't burned and our bodies needed to stay whole just like His body.)

"Don't burn the body. The Bible says it's a sin. Christina won't go to heaven. She'll burn in hell. Talk to her please. She'll listen to you. Please."

"Mom, it's the soul that goes to heaven, not the body. Her soul will not burn. Besides, it's her decision, not yours."

I was pissed. I wanted to yell, but instead I treated her like a kid. Our father had yelled enough at all of us, but especially her, to last several lifetimes.

Ene Amartea, "It's a sin," she repeated in Greek. She moaned into the phone and I wondered if Irene Pappas could do it as well as my mother. Still in Greek she said, "Did you get the letter from the priest?"

"Why would he write to me?"

"You'll see. We can't let her burn her body."

I'd stopped listening and mumbled something about having to make breakfast. I was mad but relieved that for now Christine's body remained intact. How could a dying person's wishes be dismissed so easily? Don't you get what you want in the end? If not, then when?

I hung up the phone and wondered, wasn't it enough that Christine had accepted her death? Wasn't it enough that she'd lived the way she wanted to live? Why couldn't our mother say, "Good Christine, it's good that you know what you want, good that you're deciding these things now. Good girl, my dear dying daughter."

My mom doesn't know how to comfort us but she knows what she wants for herself: fancy coffin, a pretty dress, makeup and her hair done up nice. She wants to be viewed: she's prepaid for it all and she's had the priest write out step- by step instructions for her children to follow, what to do, whom to call first (the priest), where to go. My mom's ready to ascend to heaven at a moment's notice. She's been ready for years.

Or has she? What keeps her alive at Southport Manor where she no longer wants to talk with me or anyone else on the phone? Where she sits idly and wants to do nothing? Where she waits for her *gambro* her "groom" to come take her away. Each time I visit, her heart and mind have ascended farther into unknown territories. How much longer? I think and then quickly pull back from the flame of guilt. How could I wish my mother dead?

Maybe it's like I wished my sister dead during the last months of her life. It was no life, really. But then how will I feel when I'm dying? Will I cling to each sip of water, to each kind word, to each gesture of love as if it were my last? Will I be as courageous as my sister was?

A week after Christine's death in 1999, I was at a Unity service back home. It was a cool Sunday morning in June, but I wasn't myself. I noticed the day's sermon was entitled, "Greeks Bearing Gifts." As I waited alone for the service to begin I closed my eyes and listened to the sounds around me. Directly behind I could hear a baby. The mom introduced her baby to someone as Christina. My right ear tingled like a miniature bell. Moments later I opened my eyes and turned to look. The beautiful baby had fallen asleep in a portable car seat. The mom was next to her, bright and plump. The other woman was young and pregnant. I turned and faced front, afraid I might be caught staring. Across the room sat a lone woman with curly hair and large dark sunglasses. She looked like Christine had years ago, attractive and reserved.

I looked over to my left and saw my friend Christine diagonally across from me. The top of my head radiated with warmth. Moments later after the Lord's Prayer, I ran and knelt at Christine's feet as her arms encircled my back and I was soothed by this woman who was not my mother. Later still, an attractive young biracial woman slipped into the seat next to me. My heart jumped. She could easily be my grown up daughter Alethea. This stranger looked into my eyes and smiled. I smiled back and was tempted to reach for her hand, but I didn't. The sunlight streamed across the floor and I bowed down to pray for my sister's wandering soul. I don't recall the words, only the warm energy around my heart.

Big Bad Love

I remember growing up I was taught crying was a sign of weakness. So no matter how bad or hard things got when I was raising my daughters alone, I never let them see me cry. I wanted to protect them. Money was scarce at times but I would always find a couple of bucks to put supper on the table.

I don't remember being told not to cry, but I also don't remember seeing anyone cry. I don't like having anyone watch me cry, either. The other day I was watching the movie "Wit" with Emma Thompson, who plays a lonely college professor dying of ovarian cancer. It's terribly sad. Half way into the movie, tears clogged my throat. My heart said, "Let them out," but my head responded with, "Don't cry, the kids are in the next room. They'll hear you and they'll worry." Now I wonder, was it worry or was it fear, fear of being vulnerable, of not being the strong older sister, mother and wife.

At the end of the movie, Thompson's long-ago mentor comes to visit her in the hospital. The elder woman takes off her shoes and climbs into bed alongside her former student. She puts her arms around the dying professor and reads her the children's book, *The Runaway Bunny*. In the end, the bunny gives up running and settles down with his mother.

The cuddled reading was full of love. My heart burst with its simple kindness. Wasn't this what any of us wanted when we were dying? Or alive? Wasn't this longing for love how Christine got into trouble with her new boyfriend Sal?

It was during this "going out" period that I met HIM and from now on that's how I will refer to Him. It's still real painful to say his name.

He was ruggedly handsome, had a good trade, and also owned his own place, and eventually his own business. He loved to tinker in the garage with his tools and tractors. Later he had an enormous garden he loved to tend to, all that really attracted me to him.

There was just one thing. He was a former 'Bad Boy.'

He used to do drugs, heroin back in the 60's and he did some time in prison. That didn't really bother me, we all make mistakes and that was in the past.

Something was intriguing about him – I'd never known anyone who did drugs or who was in prison.

My father and family, soon to be ex- husband, and the girls, didn't like him. I think that attracted me to him more. He was my choice.

I thought I was in Love! Still had no idea what a happy, healthy relationship was.

Now I wonder; Does anyone? Certainly our parents failed dismally. Certainly my own is a struggle simply to maintain. Certainly everyone I know is asking the same question. But still I want to scream, Why didn't you pay attention! Why didn't you leave HIM before it was too late?

One day early in the relationship I went over to his place without calling and caught him shooting drugs! I was so angry and we argued.

We didn't talk for a long time. Then one day he came over and apologized and said it would never happen again. I believed him.

HE was really pushing me to get a divorce and He didn't believe I would really do it. So to prove to him I was serious, I went to a lawyer and had divorce papers sent to Greece.

Theo came home after getting the divorce papers and was furious. Theo found out about <u>His</u> past and was really upset about the girls being around him. The girls didn't like him at all either. Theo tried to win me back, but it was too late. He said in Greece he realized me and the girls were the most important thing to him, but it was too late. I had endured too much pain.

When I resisted, Theo got real angry and started hitting me, with the girls in the house. He refused to move out, so I left. It was one of the hardest things I ever did.

The girls stayed with their father, and I went and stayed with <u>Him</u>.

I knew Theo loved the girls and would never lay a hand on them. Their ages were about 7, 9 and 10 at the time.

Theo would talk badly about me to the girls, saying I ruined his life, I broke up the family, everything was my fault, even his gambling – I drove him to it!

He finally agreed to leave and I moved back in with the girls. With everything Theo had done to me, I never spoke badly about him to the girls. He's their father, and they should respect him. Anyway I thought, they will find out on their own how he is. (The truth always comes out in the end.)

Well, I really didn't want this to become a male-bashing story but it certainly sounds like one. Looking back now it seems that starting with my father, then my husband, then "boyfriend," I was being manipulated by them – didn't realize it at the time.

I was young, vulnerable and I believed what they were telling me was the truth.

Again, I'm not saying all this stuff to make myself look good. Lord knows I have my faults.

I understood Christine's desire for love after her separation. It's as if she picked up where she left off in high school. The hidden dates, the stolen kisses, the excitement of romance. It's only now I see she was playing with fire. I wasn't to know of his drug habit until it was too late. I did know she wasn't having an easy time as a working mother.

My ex-husband's child support checks never came regularly and then stopped after awhile. He said to me, "You wanted the divorce. You support them!"

I always thought that if we divorced he would have the decency to support his kids. I guess I was wrong.

His words made me angry and made me more determined that I could do it on my own, working six days a week, at times, two jobs.

I didn't want any handouts – no welfare or food stamps, I was too proud for that.

I wanted to work for what I got.

The child support money wasn't a lot. Theo cried to the court that he wasn't making much money so he couldn't afford more. ($25 a week for each kid) But I knew the truth. He was working "under the table" a lot and the "books" only showed a portion of what he actually made. But he didn't want to give his kids even that!

That was really disturbing to me and I could not understand it! It really irks me (to this day) to see him get away with that. Looking back now I think I should have done more to make him pay up, but I was tired of fighting, arguing etc. I wanted to be free of him.

HE and I eventually lived together. I thought I was in love, but I really didn't want to get married again. Getting married the first time, I guess, left a bad taste in my mouth! Anyway I didn't feel the need to be married (probably my own way of feeling independent).

I loved working with flowers and started working in a flower shop. I took a couple of classes in floral design. I loved my work.

Christine's three girls had a hard time believing their mom had done the right thing, even though over the years they grew to love Sal. The oldest, Adriana was the same age as my birth child, Alethea, both born in 1969. Adriana was smart, headstrong and athletic. She took her homework seriously. I remember knocking on her bedroom door when she was around ten. We had just come into town. Adriana opened the door and said, "I've got too much work to do. I can come out for half an hour and then I have to get back." I was irritated and pleased at the same time. I remember thinking this girl will go far but she'll go it alone. Tina was cute, funny and popular. She loved to make us laugh with her silly faces. She was the one who got my Dad to smile. Christine named her after herself and it was Tina she felt the closest to. They looked most alike with dark hair and classic Greek noses. Kerry was beautiful, shy, and troubled. She had a tragic sadness around her large eyes even as a baby. She rarely smiled. She got into trouble early in her life and was in and out of treatment centers. Towards the end of her life, Christine tried to help her youngest by taking her in time and time again.

Adriana was the only one to have her mom's tight curly hair. She was also the one who felt she had outgrown her mother and went on to find other grown-ups to look up to, just as I had. For years we had a special relationship, and I adored her. She seemed the most like me. She seemed the most like my unknown first daughter- I would watch her and imagine my daughter doing similar things: athletics, awards, honors - both curly headed wonders. Adriana was Daddy's girl no matter how many times he broke his promises to the family. She blamed her mom for all that went wrong. (Now I wonder, did she also blame her for getting AIDS. Did she silently think: If you hadn't divorced daddy all this wouldn't have happened.) Later she put herself through college, married, became a gym teacher and bought a house. I don't know how she's doing aside from that.

Tina lived the teenage years her mother didn't have: the dances, friends, dates and clothes. She worked all through her teenage years and bought herself a new car. Tina stood by her mom until her boyfriend moved to Las Vegas to find work and she went with him several years before Christine died. Christine took that hard, partly because she always wanted to leave the east coast too.

Kerry, the youngest quit high school but later got her beautician's license like her mom had wanted to do years earlier. She started on a series of jobs that she stacked up like cups of coffee. Her large-eyed beauty got her lots of attention and boyfriends who vowed to love and take care of her forever. I don't know if she ever believed them but she sure wanted to. Her mom worried about her the most: how was she going to manage without her to fall back on? This tortured her for many years, no matter what any of us said. "She'll have to learn to live on her own without you to rescue her, she'll have to want to do better, she'll outgrow this wild phase."(Even now, years after her mom's death, Kerry's still a wanderer struggling to find her place in the world.) The wonderful thing that Kerry did provide for her mother was her first grandchild, whom Christine doted on and adored.

Despite danger signs throughout their relationship, Christine stuck with Sal.

HE was a hard worker and did excellent work- a welder. HE would talk about the future and tell me what a great life we could have together with all the money he made. HE wasn't doing drugs intravenously – I was pretty sure of that but He was taking lots of pills for a back injury. He drank his father's homemade wine daily.. smoked some pot now and then- didn't think much of it at the time. Lots of times it got out of hand. Still, I kept thinking, Things are going to get better.

I deeply regret that my daughters had to see that- he was not a very good role model.

We were together for about 10 years – almost as long as I was with my husband.

Life had its ups and downs and I took the downs in stride. He went to the hospital a few times with infections – didn't think much of it at the time. Then it seemed like all of a sudden he was acting really bizarre and strange – sometimes violent. That was something I <u>would not</u> stand for.

So I moved out and got an apartment of my own with Tina and Kerry. My oldest daughter decided to ignore everything that was going on and stayed there living with HIM.

Soon after I found out that he had a cancerous tumor in his head that caused dementia (Later learning he had AIDS.) That explained the bizarre behavior.

I really felt so sorry for him. I would go over to his place and cook and do whatever I could to help him. He deteriorated very quickly.

So many mixed emotions: I felt sad, angry, but it never dawned on me that I might be infected also.

Back in the early 80's it wasn't well known that AIDS was a sexually transmitted disease.

His brother called me one day to say that I should be checked for HIV. I was sure that the test would come out negative – I was wrong.

However much I want to damn Sal I can't seem to hang onto it for long. You see he wasn't an evil person; he wasn't a rough heartless kind of guy. And I think he truly loved my sister. The way he'd gently put his arm around her, the way he'd look at her, the way he'd dig up the earth so she could plant her tomato plants in his backyard. I don't know whether he stopped his drug habit or his drinking. I suppose once he found out he had the HIV virus he simply gave up any hopes for the future. He simply went along with the tide that was to quickly take his life. He was dead the April after Christine was diagnosed.

Throughout this whole ordeal his family was not very nice to me at all. I never did anything to those people. I felt they blamed me because I left him when he was sick.

I had so many mixed emotions. One day I would cry, the next I would be sooo angry! Would you blame me? Their son gave me a death sentence!

They were not understanding or sympathetic at all. When he died I could not bring myself to go to the funeral because of them.

The next day I went to the cemetery and placed a flower on his grave.

I've never been to Sal's grave. I suppose his family visits regularly and places flowers there. I also suppose they may still blame my sister for Sal's death. Sometimes my heart screams: It should be the other way around! It should be us blaming HIM and HIS family for Christine's death! But then another part of my heart says: What do you wish upon a guy whose already suffered and died? Why add to the misery AIDS has already brought to millions in the world?

In the midst of Christine's dying I couldn't hold onto hatreds. She needed my understanding and sympathy, and I couldn't provide that if I allowed hate to make a home in my heart. Maybe she wanted to die before me so I could take care of her, so I could give her the love she needed to move on ahead. But then it wasn't only me who gave her love. It was never only me. Christine had her daughters, Christine had her grandson and she had our mother and brothers who stopped by with gifts of money and food. Most of all she had her last romantic love, her guardian angel, Andy, who called countless times every day, who stopped by with her favorite foods, videos and flowers. He stood by her until her last breath. There is no greater gift one love can give another. Christine was surrounded by people who cared.

Why then do I hesitate to include them, to give them just as large a role in her death as in her life? I don't know, I only know that I'm possessive of her death unlike her life.

Maybe protective is a better word. Maybe there wasn't enough understanding and sympathy to go around. No one wanted to accept her eventual death – it was too painful. Maybe the miles made it less so: I didn't have to be there to watch her wither away. But then couldn't I have pushed away her death? Couldn't I have pretended she had longer than she did?

I couldn't. Not as the oldest, not as the one who was supposed to know more, when all the while I was just trying to catch up. Trying to catch up to where she had run to ahead of me. I was scared. Scared shit-less. What did I know about death?

Weeks after my sister died I was up in my bedroom with the door closed. The air conditioning was on high but I couldn't cool my body down. I was reading an Alaskan memoir hoping the images of snow and ice would bring cool thoughts. The flames of hell would never burn in Alaska. I imagined Christine's body in the casket about to be wheeled into the inferno, the fires which so terrified my mother. But first I was back at the funeral to take one last look. One last look at the long flowered dress Andy had chosen. She was covered from the waist down with her purple and maroon lap blanket. Close to her heart lay a white and golden angel doll that had the same Mona Lisa smile I had so loved on my sister. My heart didn't allow me to go in that place where her body would be destroyed. Terror lay there. How would the ashes look? Would there be colors? Would there be anything recognizable?

The bedroom air stood still. The temperature escalated. I didn't remember ever feeling so hot. Was it the degrees or was it the image of my sister's body burning? My heart was on fire.

Now, in the late fall of 2001, my heart aches to cool those flames of memory. It jumps to a happier time when

Christine was barely alive but laughing over something her grandson had done.

"Connie this is so funny. One day Mikey's over and I'm not feeling so good. I put on a Barney video, but he only wants to follow me around. My stomach's a mess so I run to the bathroom but don't close the door in case he needs me. He follows and watches me throw up like he has so many other times. Suddenly he crouches over just like me, opens his mouth and makes a gagging noise and says, 'Look Grandma I can throw up good too!' He's so adorable I just wanted to squeeze him to pieces!"

I watched Christine chuckle. At first I was shocked – how could throwing up be funny? How could this be good for the child? But then I saw this little kid loving his grandma so much that he'd play any game she made up for him. What could I do but laugh? Just then I looked over at my too thin sister and remember watching a Slim-Fast commercial together. Christine started talking to the screen, something I do too.

"All these girls want to lose weight. Well I've got the fool-proof plan for you girls – just get AIDS! You'll lose all the weight you want! Guaranteed!"

I didn't know how to react to this either. It felt like she was putting a hex on people. But then I said, Hey, let her be pissed! Let her be pissed at those who will live on in ignorance. At those who will live when she is long gone: her mother, her brothers, her children and her sister.

Now whenever I see a billboard or magazines of skinny women, images of dying emaciated faces transpose themselves on the new "after diet" smiling pretty ones staring out into nothing. Wouldn't the dying skeletal bodies love to have those "before diet" features of too full faces, breasts and thighs? Wouldn't they wish for ample rolls of life in the flesh? Why does death, like life, demand such an abundance of time and space?

114

If only I could always believe Dr. Elizabeth K
Ross's words:

*Death is the key to the door to life. It is the denial of
death that is partially responsible for people living empty,
purposeless lives; for when you live as if you'll live forever,
it becomes too easy to postpone the things you know you
must do.*

I re-read these handwritten words taped above my
computer and ask: How can death be the key to the door to
life? How can being reminded of death keep me truly alive?
Maybe knowing we will die–I will die–becomes the opening
through which I can emerge as a more honest and present
human being. Christine's dying created a deeper realization
that Yes, I too will follow, and that I cannot continue to
postpone expressing my love, writing my pages and living
like there will be always be a tomorrow. For it's this I know
for sure: Christine's death unlocked my long- forgotten soul.
I imagine our sister spirits as warm pillows of sand at the
seashore with gentle tears flowing freely between us.

Sudden Death

I think there are two kinds of people in a sense: Those who live life to its fullest and those who merely exist. Would you rather have 10 glorious years living or 70 years merely existing?

It's Thanksgiving morning. I awaken with a start – before the birds and before the sun. I've been dreaming about Christine. I get up, put on my robe and go downstairs to make coffee and sit. I see the large purple journal with Christine's photo glued on the front. I stare at her pleasing profile among the lushness of the trees and bushes behind her. Her hair is long and fluffy and she's wearing sunglasses. She's got that Mona Lisa smile and a bright pink shirt on. I open the book to a blank page and remember the dream. I'm running around giving speeches in large auditoriums. I see Christine by my right shoulder – slightly behind me – very patient and quiet. She's waiting for me to finish so we can go on to the next engagement. I close my eyes and wait for more but instead the image disappears. Just like that. Why is Christine watching me? Is she trying to tell me something? If so what might that be?

Hours later we're getting ready to go out for Thanksgiving dinner at Michael's mom's house. But before that we make a quick stop to see his cousin Dale in the hospital. He and his wife always celebrated the holidays with us, and Thanksgiving is his favorite time of year. I want to take him Mika's pumpkin pie and Jason's get well banner.

Michael's younger cousin had open- heart surgery two days ago. Everyone's nervous but reassured. If anyone's going to make it out of that surgery it'd be healthy, trim, daily jogger, handsome Dale. Still I want to see his face for myself. Michael drives us to Northwestern Hospital in downtown Chicago. Because there's no parking available, Michael stays with the car and I gather up my things.

"Mom, Jason's fallen asleep. Should we wake him or should you and me go on upstairs?"

"Let's leave him Mika. You know how he gets when someone wakes him up." At that Jason jumps up abruptly and opens the car door, "I want to go too! Don't leave me behind. I want to hold the balloon, give me the balloon for Dale."

"Jason, let Mika carry it; you've got the banner and here's the masking tape you can carry too so we can hang it up. He'll like the sign you made." He takes the tape and we walk into the lobby. It's like we've walked into the Ritz Carlton hotel, the rich leather couches, the elegant paintings in a large open space.

"Wow, this is some place, Mom, where do they hide the elevators?"

"Let's check at the desk."

A large friendly receptionist gives us visitor's badges and directs us to the left and around a wall. We take the elevator; stop at 14, and the kids run to the floor- to- ceiling window and look out. Everything looks so small and insignificant. Mika says to us, "If the glass breaks and we fall, we'd die. Don't stand too close to the window. How come Dale's so high up?"

"This is a fancy hospital and he's lucky to have such a view," I say, "Maybe he knows somebody who works here. Let's find his room." We take a right turn and at the end of the hall find 1426. We quietly walk in.

"Linda, Happy Thanksgiving."

"Come on in," says Linda. "Buddy's been waiting for you, he's hungry. And Dale's tired but all right."

"Honey the kids and Connie are here."

I'm relieved to see Dale with his glasses on watching the football game. He's pale, but still looks like himself.

"We brought you some stuff," I say.

Jason and Mika crowd the bed. "Hi Dale. We want to hang up your banner." Jason tries to unravel the sign by himself. "Boy this room doesn't have much in it!"

I look around to find a good spot to put my basket of flowers. I hold onto them for a few moments and then lay them down on a small table on the other side of the bed. Linda, Mika, and I help Jason with the banner that says, *Get Well Soon* and has little notes from the four of us.

Linda points out the one that says, there's a pot of rice waiting for Dale at our house and we all laugh. Dale's known for eating mass quantities of rice. The banner is on the wall directly in front of his bed and over a large, dark painting. It brightens the room. His dad, Buddy, who's visiting from California, nods in our direction and puts on his jacket. He's ready to go with us.

"Dale, when you get home we'll bring over some food. Michael's got a new outdoor cooker he wants to fry a turkey in, so you can have turkey next week. How's that?"

"Good. I can't eat now; I'm tired and only want to sleep."

We all stand for a moment not saying anything. Jason and Mika don't know what to do with a sick Dale. They're used to horsing around with him.

"If you change your mind about some food, call us and we'll drop some by later on this afternoon," I say to Linda.

"You've brought so much already," Linda says. I look at her and smile. Linda compliments Dale's good looks with looks of her own. She has a cute figure, beautiful skin and large attractive eyes. They've been married for 9 years and they're still very much in love. I can tell by the way they hang on to each other

"Oh, Linda here's a book I thought you might like, *My Dream of You* by the Irish journalist O'Faolain. It's about a writer, forbidden romance and a best friend's sudden death.

It's wonderful. And here's a new magazine, 'Real Simple' that you might like."

"Thanks Connie, you read good books so I'm sure I'll like it."

I reach over to give Dale a kiss but the bed stand is in the way and he puts his hand up and says, "Oh you don't have to kiss me – it's all right." I take my right hand and put it on his hair and forehead. We look at each other deeply and then the moment is gone forever.

"Let's go," I say but both Jason and Mika are already headed for the hallway. They turn to say, "Bye!"

We leave with Buddy who's walking very slowly. Michael is waiting for us downstairs. We get in and the ride north on Lakeshore Drive is unusually quiet.

(Weeks later Jason will tell me his worries while in Dale's hospital room. "Mom, when I looked over at Dale's machine I was so scared it was going to stop working and I couldn't get that out of my mind. That's all I could think about in the car. I didn't want to tell anyone. I was so afraid.")

Mika has brought her knitting and she's determined to finish the sock hat she started last week. Michael has the excuse of driving and Buddy stares out into the gray Lake on our right. I'm behind him, and as I watch the back of his head I wonder how worried he is. He's eighty-four and has had several heart surgeries himself. Dale didn't want him to come but he came anyway. The Lake is choppy and uninviting. I'm glad we're inside the warm car heading to Michael's moms for a delicious dinner.

Two hours later Dale collapses while on his way to the bathroom. No resuscitation measures by the nurses and doctors will save him. Within moments he is dead. His wife screams but nothing will bring him back.

My heart shouts, This doesn't make sense! How could a perfectly healthy man die without warning? No one is prepared. Dale, least of all, I'm afraid. With Christine I had time to get used to the idea of her death. Christine had time to get used to the idea of her death. Everything about Dale promised a successful recovery. What happened?

The next day Linda said his last words were that he felt full. I try to give meaning to these words. Maybe his life was as full as it was going to get and he sensed he was ready to move on? Or maybe he sensed his body was too full to carry him any farther? Or maybe he had no idea what would happen next. The last maybe is the one that scares me the most, the not knowing what will happen next. How could he not have time to prepare? How could he not get his good-byes in? How could he die not knowing?

Later that day after the shock and tears, I tell Jason and Mika that Christine will take care of Dale. Later still, someone says he died because there was a place available at the table in heaven. Another much older relative asks how come there wasn't a place available for her yet. Another says, "Oh, nobody wants you at the table – you're too ornery!" I like this idea of Dale's seat at the table in heaven with Christine hovering about making sure he's got all that he needs. (She'd met Dale years earlier and like every other woman, thought he was a hunk.) Christine was good at taking care of other's needs, much of the time before her own. Dale was good at taking care of his own needs and aside from his beloved wife, he didn't have to worry about others. He had a good job, made good money, traveled and did what he pleased. Was Dale ready without knowing he was ready? How do we reconcile with his sudden disappearance?

Sometimes I wish I had the kind of faith that was solid, the kind that rarely doubted or questioned. The morning of Christine's funeral several years earlier was one such time. I doubted everything, why the sun came out, why the beach was still there, why I felt naked even though I was dressed in black from top to bottom. I felt raw. A part of my heart will always remain at the funeral home in East Haven where I last saw my sister's body, where I cried between my mother and younger brother as we sat in the front row listening to two very different speakers. The sweet handsome Greek priest prayed over someone he didn't really know and really didn't approve of – her divorce, her lover, her AIDS, her cremation wishes. He was there to soothe my mother's aching heart. He was there to give a religious pardon for her life and death as a baptized Christian. It felt generic; Christine had stopped going to church long ago.

The second speaker was Dr. Nancy Angoff who knew my sister well. It was this Jewish doctor who captured the essence of Christine's courageous journey into death. It was this doctor from another religion who knew what most people in front of her didn't know, that Christine had become more of her true self during the eight years she lived with the virus than at any other time in her life. During those eight years she identified her wishes to travel and to live peacefully by the beach; she made medical decisions about her care, and she lived a life full of gentle love until her dying day. The doctor spoke for twenty minutes about this patient who had changed her life, who had taught her how to be a more compassionate and caring physician and human being. I remember wondering if others in the room recognized the beauty of my sister's journey; if they recognized my sister in the courageous light that was now being shed upon her. For many she might remain the "poor Christine" of long ago, whose death only solidified her bad luck, her early ascent into adulthood and death.

By the close of the service my heart was bursting with sorrow I could no longer contain. I turned to the thirty or so people behind me and suddenly announced, "Christine was the bravest person I know. She lived the best way she knew how. She was a wonderful person. Someday, someday I will write a book about her. Someday you will read about how brave my sister was."

I struggled to say more but my mom was tugging at my jacket sleeve. Was she trying to console me? Was she going to collapse? She continued to pull and I turned to look at her red lips as she whispered, *Popsi Tora*, or "Stop now," and then, "Don't forget to tell them to come and eat, tell them where the restaurant is. Don't forget to tell Father before he leaves. Don't forget."

I stared at my mother's face and I didn't know what I was supposed not to forget. I stared as if I'd been stung by a quick hand across my cheek. Her face was impatient with me. There was too much rouge and lipstick all over it. Her mouth was open, her eyes on fire. Was she angry with me, embarrassed, or just impatient to get on with things? To have all this misery behind her only to realize she had outlived her younger daughter? I recuperated quickly and did as my mother said. I announced the invitation and offered directions to the seafood restaurant by the water. The sweet priest came with us, but Dr. Angoff had to get back to work.

I don't know if my mother's misery over her daughter's death continues. Her heart and soul have always been hers and hers alone. She doesn't share much of that journey with others. To her strangers have always been anyone outside the immediate family, but now I wonder if those of us inside have also always remained strangers.

It's this wondering I often pack with me whenever I journey out east. Five weeks after Dale's death in 2001 I was on a plane headed east to visit my mom. It was the day after Christmas, Christine's 50th birthday. Minutes before boarding, I had read a *Sun-Times* article about a woman named Christine who'd snatched a sixteen month- old baby girl from the Greyhound bus station. I wondered if Christine had been anywhere near the bus station today, maybe picking out a birthday present for herself, someone to keep her company. (Days later the baby was found unharmed. The woman's name wasn't Christine after all.) I stared into the sky hoping to see my sister's face. Suddenly the young girl next to the window pulled down the shutter and we were in darkness. I wanted to say something about enjoying the sunlight but I didn't. The girl turned on the overhead light and opened up a thick textbook. She started to underline paragraphs with a yellow marker. I pulled out my novel for book group and hoped I could get further into this Joyce

Carol Oates novel, *We Were the Mulvaneys*. She wasn't one of my favorite authors but I was enjoying the story's narrator, who's a writer looking back and trying to understand what's happened to his once happy family. Every now and then I peaked over at the girl and saw she hadn't turned a page. Eventually she fell asleep with the yellow marker still in her right hand.

Four hours later I walked into my mom's nursing home in Southport, just about ten miles from where I grew up in Bridgeport. I found her by the bedroom door, stooped over in a sofa chair wearing large dark sunglasses.

"Connie, is you?" she said. You make me a surprise. Good. You got feta cheese?"

"Feta, olives and fresh bread." I bent down and gave her a kiss on the cheek. "I also have some spanikopita Mika made for you. She loved laying out the filo dough, and she loves the crusty edges just like we all do," I said hoping to further connect my ten- year old Asian daughter to her largely unknown Greek Yiayia.

"Really? Good, I'm glad Mika likes our pita. What about Jason?"

"He's not crazy about it. He doesn't like the spinach or the white cheese; he only likes broccoli and yellow American cheese. Michael likes it though," I said.

"How come Jason can't like it? Tell him to try again. Michael is good man. Give me feta and bread now."

I take out the paper plates I've brought and use my hands to cut off a piece of feta.

"Don't you have a knife to cut the cheese? You should always carry a small little knife you don't know when you need it."

"You can't bring even small knives on the plane with you anymore. Ever since September 11th the airlines are very strict. No scissors, not even nail clippers!" I didn't mention the body scanning, the police, the dogs, the lines or the anger I felt at the strangers who had taken away the simplicity of travel. I didn't want to remind my mother of the unsafe world we lived in. Why worry an old lady? I put a napkin on her lap and handed her a hunk of bread along with the plate of olives and feta. I stared at her face and still saw my mother. I was relieved. Each time I visited I was afraid she wouldn't recognize me or I wouldn't recognize her. Her hair was colored differently, a red-brown, and it was teased back from her face. I couldn't see her eyes behind the tinted glasses she didn't want to remove. She was wearing a blue cotton housedress and a white sweater. Her body was bent over her plate and her large swollen hands took the food slowly.

I sat on her bed and we ate in silence. I turned to look at her roommate, Angie who was asleep by the window. She was bedridden and slept most of the day. No one came to visit Angie. She'd never married or had children and only had a doctor nephew who ten years ago had dropped her off along with a new Sony color television. The Sony broke and her nephew never returned. I brought her flowers whenever I visited and this time it was a white poinsettia, which I'd left on her nightstand. I couldn't imagine not having company from the outside.

I turned to my mom and gave her more cheese and bread. In a bit I said, "Today's Christine's birthday. She's fifty today. Remember how she hated being born the day after Christmas and only getting one present? Maybe we can go out with Jim and Tas and celebrate with some fried clams and wine."

"I can't believe it. I can't believe it. I think she comes to visit me one day. I can't believe she's dead," my mom said in a whisper. She reached her hand out and I held it with both of mine. It was warm, but rough. She didn't mention the birthday or going out to celebrate with my brothers.

"She's been gone over two years but it's like she never left." My heart sank deeper into my chest. How did my mother manage to keep her heartbreak in check? Had she buried the tears along with all her other heartbreaks, or were the tears on the surface, waiting to engulf her? How did a mother bury her child and live?

"Do you want to try the pita?"

"Just a small piece, I can't eat too much."

I handed her a corner square and she took a bite.

"Oh, Connie it's good."

"Mika's learned to work fast with the filo before it dries out. I tell her about how you and Yiayia used to spend all day making the dough from scratch and how you'd start early in the morning with your aprons and head scarves on and how you were afraid hairs would get into the spinach mix." I took her empty plate, and said, "I'll save the rest for tomorrow."

Her quilted bed was now our table, our home. My family's household had disappeared and what my mother still possessed fit in a nightstand, a chest drawers and a small closet against the wall. I walked over to the nightstand and found unopened mail stuffed into several of the drawers. I scooped up the letters and began to rip them open. Christmas cards, get well cards, thinking of you cards from her brother, nephew, niece, grand- children and me.

"How come you haven't opened your mail? Look, the kids sent you this Halloween card and you've got a bunch of holiday cards too."

My mom didn't say anything as I looked at each one and read them to her, something she used to beg me to do in the past.

"Connie, read this card to me again, please, I like to hear the words."

"Oh mom not now, maybe later, anyway I already read it, don't you remember what it says?"

Now her hands didn't even reach out to hold the cards I tried to give her.

"Put away for later, put away. I don't want to see. I can't look now."

My mom's world was reduced to what she could put on her lap. I ached at the loss, but also considered the simplicity in this- no yesterday, no tomorrows, only the *now* of the present moment. Wasn't this what I too was striving for, the presence of being in the moment? Yes, the gift of today without worrying about the past or the future. But then

I suddenly wondered, Can a writer write without a past and a future?

The next day my brothers and I took my mom to Jimmie's seafood restaurant in West Haven to eat clams and be close to Christine. Many of her ashes were scattered just beyond our table window by the large boulder in the water. The gray choppy water was uninviting and I worried over how cold my sister used to get during these dark months. After dinner we got in the car and stopped nearer the boulder. I stared into the vast seascape and asked my mother, "Why don't you say a prayer for Christine now that we're here?"

"I can't pray to water. I don't think it's right." she said quietly with her head bowed down.

Would the church or the priest object to praying over ashes? Was my mother afraid of doing something sacrilegious? I tossed aside the question suddenly irritated at my mother's reluctance to soothe us, her remaining children, her reluctance to acknowledge the spirit of her second daughter. I got out of the car and walked closer to the water. My younger brother came with me. My other brother was behind the wheel and stayed with our mother.

Tassie and I stood alone on the smaller rocks as the wind pulled at our coats and pants. He was much taller than I. His bearded face was younger and still handsome. Tas is an artist who paints wonderful canvases when his heart and mind are united. When they are not united it's difficult for him to live and work. I looked around and imagined the warmer weather when pathways were filled with people walking and talking, when older Italian men played bocce, when children ran to catch up with their kites. This was a place Christine loved to walk along with Andy.

"Tas, I think Christine's here. A lot of her ashes are here. There must be some part of her spirit here, don't you think?"

"I don't know. I hope so, but she hated this kind of day, so I don't know if she's somewhere else now,

126

someplace warmer. I can't imagine her sticking around here for long."

"Maybe you're right. Maybe she's someplace warmer like Florida. Let's say a prayer anyway. I brought the one on her prayer card. I'll read that."

"Let me say the Lord's Prayer first."

We took each other's gloved hands and recited both prayers. We waited for a response, but the only one we got was the cry of the hungry seagulls overhead. The cold had numbed my cheeks.

Did my mom already know what Christine's favorite poem knew? That she would remain forever all around us? That the unspoken words were already embedded on our hearts? Just then I was reminded of several lines from her favorite poem,

> *Do not think of me and cry*
> *I am not dead; I did not die*
> *Think of me and I will be there.*
> *Don't think of me and cry*
> *I am not dead. I did not die.*

The words lingered and congregated at the far off crease where the sky and water unite. I imagined the crease might be a comfortable spot to rest. We both turned at the same time and headed back to the waiting car.

Several days later it was time for me to leave for the airport, a moment I've always hated. I was full of guilt over leaving my mother behind to fend for herself. But this time was a little different. I turned to say my good-byes, but my mother beat me to it. First she removed her tinted glasses, looked up at me from her chair and stared into my eyes. Then she said,

"When you come is good but when you leave is hard. I'm not gonna let you go. I'm not gonna let you get on the airoplane."

"I know Mom, I wish I was closer so I could see you more," I said realizing I didn't used to mean this. I used to crave the distance as if that would make me less like my mother. Now I imagined myself coming twice a week to open her mail, comb her hair and iron her wrinkled house-dresses.

"I can't express, I can't express how much I love you. I'm no good with words, but I love you – I love you so much. I'm sorry I can't express so good."

Our eyes locked into a steady gaze and my heart soared. I didn't know what to say. My mother saw me. She recognized who I was. Suddenly I wondered why I'd spent most of my life doubting her love. We'd never shared the same language between her broken English and my broken connection. Maybe we had always been linked in a world without language, in a time before words. My heart felt light and wet as I knelt down in front of her chair and put my arms around her waist. She put her hands gently on my back and we were together. I touched her cheeks with my lips. Then I quickly got up, turned to leave and didn't look back. It's a moment I take with me everywhere now. It's a moment I share with Christine as she perches on my right shoulder and waits for me to finish living in my dream.

Lucky to Be Alive

Feel this great sense of calmness. I know everything will be O.K. Everything will fall into place. Just let things happen naturally. Feel absolutely no anger any more. I want the people who care about me to be around. For years I have been praying to God to <u>please help me.</u> Whatever it takes. Not necessarily not to die – to show me the way – to cope? To? Just <u>help me</u>. My prayers have been answered.

Despite Christine's increasing weakness she was determined to live one day at a time. Her bravest months, her dying months were filled with activity. Watching her red- haired grandson Mikey most weekday mornings, taking rides along the sound, spending quiet days on the beach between trips to Chicago and Las Vegas.

Oct. 1998: Went for another ERCP procedure at Yale. Everything went OK. Halloween is coming up. I like decorating the house, the spookiness of it all. It was always a fun time for me. It's hard to describe how I feel lately – the word 'numb' best describes it. Don't want to think too much – about the past, or anything. Life's too short. Why waste time worrying?

Life is short but how do we get ourselves to stop worrying? The other night I dreamt everyone was still alive, my dad and Christine along with my mom, my two brothers and me. The six of us are in our old house on State Street. My father sits at the head of the table in the dining room smiling. My mom stands with her back to us. The four grown-up kids are huddled in the cramped front hallway. I remember thinking in my dream: I want us all to be together again. Suddenly I say, "Hey, let's go buy some maple walnut ice cream!" My brother Jim says, "That's a good idea, but where at this hour?" Christine and Tas don't say anything but their bodies move closer to ours. My parents shout their approval as if I've just won them another chance at life, at being together, at happiness.

In my dream, a gallon of maple walnut ice cream suddenly appears. Maple walnut is my family's favorite kind of ice cream. Our plastic spoons dig into the cardboard container: the smooth taste of maple mixes with a hint of coffee and the fat wet walnuts tease the tongue with their woody flavor.

The only dream I ever remember Christine talking about was the one she had right after one of her hospital stays. This time it was for severe pancreatic problems. Most of her medicine was stopped and she was put on new pain medication that knocked her out. Later, after her death, I'd find she'd written about this dream along with other entries on a yellow legal sized notepad.

Thursday evening, March 12,1998: Everyone was asleep. I woke up, my heart racing. I was shaky. I'll try to explain it. I was lying on the floor holding Mikey. I saw myself looking at me from above, telling everyone I loved them - Mom, Connie, Tina, Kerry. I heard the most beautiful music. It was beckoning me to walk toward it. My mother was calling to me, saying if I leave I won't come back here, I'll be somewhere else. So I told her yes, I will be back. That instant, my eyes flew open. A dream? Maybe. Never had one like that before. Out of body experience? A spiritual awakening? A revelation? It was more than a dream.

I got up, got some water to drink, sat in the living room where Connie was sleeping; thought she might wake up, but she was fast asleep and I didn't want to wake her. I found myself afraid to go back to sleep, afraid I wasn't going to wake up if I did. Finally about 4 a.m. I fell asleep. I remember thinking, Wait a minute, I can't die now, I was going to have fried clams on Friday. Dr. Angoff was coming to visit on Friday night, No, no I couldn't go yet.

I recall thinking, well maybe it would be a good time to go now. Connie & Tina are both here, it would be convenient. I would die & that would be an end to their suffering somewhat. "It's over, let's go home and that's it." An END NOW – If I don't go now, the suffering will linger. Make it worse?? For everyone??

I can't go now...Connie's 50th birthday is coming up...Tina's Las Vegas wedding is coming up in May.. I don't want to spoil their plans to celebrate them.

How can a death ever be convenient? My heart lightens at the idea of fried clams keeping her alive! A couple of Sundays a year my father would drive us down to Savin Rock in West Haven to eat fried clams at Phyllis's. Recently my brothers reminded me that as a child, Christine didn't like them and got my father to order her a hamburger instead. I wish now I could ask her when she started liking clams.

I remember Christine's excitement the next morning in telling us the dream that was more than a dream. Was it the new pain- killers she was on? Was it a premonition of what was to come? More than anything else Christine wanted to know if it was real. She told the dream many times over the next few days. I got scared. Oh, God is this the beginning of the end? Is this IT?

On that Friday we did have fried clams, only by then Christine couldn't keep any food down for long. Dr. Angoff came to visit that evening. We were huddled together with Christine in her living room, Andy, Tina, Tas, Kerry and I wanting the doctor to tell us how much longer our sister, mother, lover had to live.

"What's going to happen to my mom and what does the dream she just told you about mean?" Tina asked.

"She's been through a lot. Maybe the dream means she has more living to do. Mikey has given her so much pleasure," Dr. Angoff said. "Christine, everyone's here because they love you and want to be with you. Just take it a day at a time. No one knows what the future holds for any of us."

"I'm all right. I don't feel any pain and I'm sleeping better. I got scared that my dream meant I was going to die soon, but then Mom pulled me back. So, Doctor, you're right I'm not ready to go yet!" Christine said.

I was afraid Christine would die before my fiftieth birthday two months later and Tina's wedding a month after that. I also remember talking with Tina and wondering if she should postpone it. Tina was already married the previous Thanksgiving. My Mom and I had arranged for a small wedding in the Greek Church in Bridgeport so Christine could see her daughter a happy bride.

"This bigger Las Vegas wedding is for us in our new home. I don't know what to do."

"I can't very well put off my birthday! I could postpone our trip to Hawaii this summer, but what if Christine lives for years to come? What if by some miracle she gets to live? Won't it seem silly then to have put our lives on hold?" I said.

"Whatever we do it'll seem like the wrong thing without my mom around. Dad says he's coming but you know how he is. I won't believe it till I see him walking through the door. Mom's too weak right now to make the trip. Nobody can handle this. Kerry and Andy are basket cases and God knows what's going through Adriana's head. I don't get it. I'll never get it," Tina said.

"I can't believe we're talking this way! Worried about stupid stuff when your mom needs us and we're so far away. She's the last person on earth who should have more troubles put on her. Maybe in her next life she'll have it easy. I hope to God she does come back to live a long life as a happy woman."

Just as I'm typing "long life" a flash of Christine's words about growing old makes me sit straighter in my chair. I search for the entry on that yellow notepad.

Mar '99: Waiting to catch my car ride back home from the clinic on a breezy March day- waiting inside the hallway, I see them, older women getting out of work at the hospital. Gee, I think to myself, she's got to be at least 65 or 70 years old, dressed nicely, hair neatly done, scurrying about, running to catch their rides back home. That one looks much older, then I thought to myself, **I wonder how I would look if I had gotten the chance to grow old?** *'Look at them practically running at 'their age!'*

Today made it more definite. Decided to check into Hospice soon, even for a couple of months. I need to rest, not to worry and be as comfortable as possible. I feel myself getting weaker all the time.

My head spins with Christine's lost possibility. What would she have looked like had she grown old naturally? My brother Jimmy recently told me something a friend had said about taking a long time to die: *We die in pieces.* Certainly that was true for my dad, my mom and my sister. Is it also true of us three remaining siblings? Of most people still living?

The other day I was talking with Bram and mentioned this "Dying in pieces."

"Don't we also *Live in pieces*?" he said. And I thought, Of course we do. We live and die in pieces, not unlike the pieces torn from old clothing and sewn into patchwork quilts, quilts that will outlast us all.

Yesterday I read a review of a new book called, *If I Live to be 100*, stories of people who have made it to 100. Why couldn't she have made it to at least 50? How long will I live? My Unity friend Christine who wants to make it to 100 has got about 15 years to go. She looks marvelous. I'll be 55 soon. How do I look? I'd like to think a bit like Irene

Pappas, the Greek star of Zorba fame: dark hair, deep eyes and a tongue on fire.

In a way the years seem like an eternity: 55, 56, 57, 58, 59, 60, 61, 62, 63, 64, 65, 66, 67, 68, 69, 70, 71, 72, 73, 74, 75, 76, 77, 78, 79, 80, 81, 82, 83, 84, 85, 86, 87, 88, 89, 90, 91, 92, 93, 94, 95, 96, 97, 98, 99, 100.

In another way they seem like a forty-five minute trip to pick up some ice cream, as rapid as heartbeats.

Sometimes I wish I didn't have this nagging urge to make sense of my life with words. At other times I only wish the words would come easier.

There is nothing easy about reading Christine's entry on Wednesday, May 19, 1999, one month before she will die.

Here I am at Hospice. Actually it's real nice. My room is comfortable; the people are very caring and nice. Good feeling pampered, really don't have to worry about a thing. Living from day to day, trying not to think about the future.

I'm so lucky to have Connie and Andy, they are so good to me.

Kerry and Mikey are going to visit today...

I remember Christine and I getting dressed on the day of our father's funeral in 1988. My father hadn't wanted to die; he wasn't ready. He wasn't used to letting go of anything. He thought if he could hang on long enough, death might pass him by, almost like a staring contest or an eating contest- he always won at those.

Christine and I were in my parent's bedroom, fixing our hair and putting on make-up at the large mirror attached to the bureau. We caught a reflection of each other in the glass and our expression froze for a moment.

"God Connie, here we are worrying about our looks and Pop is dead! What does it matter what we look like?"

I didn't say anything at first, sensing she was right. I picked up the red blush and applied some color to my pale cheeks anyway. It was only May and I hadn't gotten any sun color yet. I felt like an albino. "We can't not look in the mirror," I said.

"You're right. Our faces have to shine a little so we won't look dead, ourselves. These all- black clothes make me feel creepy." Christine said.

I looked at my sister in the mirror and suddenly wondered which one of us would die first. I pushed away this unwelcome fear of death by telling myself it would be a long, long way off. I imagined us growing old – really old – together reminiscing and laughing on the beach in long flowing caftans and large sun hats, with all the time in the world.

Years later I was at a smaller mirror, alone this time. I was getting dressed for the funeral. I had on black loose pants and an oversized black jacket. I was gelling my hair and trying to get it to poof up when I started to cry. What the fuck was I doing fixing my hair in front of Christine's bathroom mirror? The same mirror in which she had stared at herself countless times, wondering how such a sunken face could be repaired. Now I wondered the same thing. How could I ever repair this sunken mess of tears that set so heavily on my cheeks? Where was my sister? Weren't we supposed to have buried my mother first? Together? Why was the order so messed up? I pulled at the roots of my hair roughly and the pain soothed my aching heart.

It is springtime and with it holds the promise of new Life. Yesterday's pain and hardships are over, gone forever. It is time to begin anew. (May 1999)

I remember the last day of my sister's life. It was Father's Day of 1999. I had this last thing to do for my younger sister, help her die a peaceful death. Later that day she would become the leader, upsetting the order, an order I thought had been set at birth. The sun was shining, the birds were chirping, but Christine was a cord of wood unable to move or speak.

135

I'd spent the last couple of nights in her room on a rollaway bed. I sat by her bed, holding her hand and waiting. Sometimes I spoke; sometimes I didn't. It was too late for words, anyhow, just like Christine had said. It was still not too late for her eldest daughter to appear, but she won't. She is stubborn, like my father. Age has softened my stubbornness, but she is still young and oh so righteous.

I sat and held onto my aching love and wondered where it would go after my sister had died. This was the first death I'd witnessed up close.

I ached to know why love is so difficult, so elusive, so tragic not unlike the Greeks of ancient times, had so little changed since then? My heart fluttered around my sister's room like the cardinal at the window watching us. This time we were inside the display case, locked inside our humanness; the cardinals free to roam.

I let go of my sister's cold hand and walked out to find a nurse. I talked with Mary and she told me I needed to give Christine permission to let go, to release her from this earthly life. My heart cried out, No I don't want to! But my heart also knew there was no one else who could do this last thing for her. It was a kindness I could not refuse. I walked back into the room and saw Christine hadn't moved a muscle. I stood over her and whispered in her ear, "It's me, Connie. I'm right here with you. I'm going to talk. Please let me know if you can hear me. I need to know if you can hear me." I sat and waited for a sign. Within moments Christine's eyes opened for a few seconds and she looked deeply into mine for the last time. Her eyes were large and dark. An ocean of time lay behind them. I stared into her and she slowly closed them, as if the effort to keep them open was too much. I began to talk.

"Christine, it's all right to let go. There's nothing left for you to do here; you've done it all. You've given birth to three beautiful children and you've spent time with your grandchild who will always remember you as his Yiayia. You didn't do anything wrong. You lived the best way you knew how. You've said you're good-byes. Your oldest won't be coming, but it's not your fault. It's not your fault; it's not your fault. Let her go along with the others. They will all be fine."

I stopped and put my head down by her chest. She was still breathing. The silence around us felt holy. I start again, "It's Sunday, it's Father's Day. It's a beautiful sunny day, perfect for a picnic. Remember how Pop would make shish-ka-bob on the grill at the beach? Imagine us all at Seaside Park, happy again. He'll be there cooking and Teta Lena and Katina will be there too and all our families. They're just waiting for your arrival. Let them take you with them. They'll treat you well. They'll treat you like the time at your baptism, remember? The time you were the princess in your frilly white dress and curly hair. Only this time it will be forever. Go on ahead."

I stopped and put my head back down by her chest. My words were gone. My heart felt suspended and outside my body, as if I could watch it from afar, pumping on its own. The hollow space under my chest was vacant. I was exhausted. I only wondered when the others would arrive.

Soon Andy and two good friends arrived. The four of us sat at each end of the bed, protecting the edges of her existence. Andy put on peaceful ocean music and Joan read some of her favorite poetry. Katherine was quiet, maybe not knowing how an elder greets the death of one so much younger. I was thankful to these three strangers who had became family to my sister and to me

At four ten that afternoon Christine died. It was peaceful, just the way she had wanted it. The four of us sat with her for a while before we called the nurse in. My duty to my younger sister was almost done. I didn't want to leave the room where I had spent so many hours with her. I didn't want to leave her body alone; it didn't feel right. We slowly packed and then I sat some more. How could it be over just like that? I'd had years being the older sister and I would never let that part of me go. I would always have my sister with me just like she had always had me with her. She remained in my heart and there we settled in as Sea Sisters Forever.

Thank God, throughout my life I had my sister Connie to look up to. She and I have gotten really close. She understands me better than anyone and it's been good sharing similar thoughts and feelings, long talks on the phone. I really admire her, always have. I always thought she was the smartest one of us all for leaving this damned place. Too many bad memories here.
I admire her courage and strength for saying and doing what she wanted or needed to at the time. She always stood up to my father or anyone (I never could) and spoke her mind. I really admire that. The way she lives her life, always wanting to better herself, going to school, reading a lot, being outgoing, having lots of friends, being a great mom for her kids, the list goes on and on: Her generosity, her open heart, always giving of herself. I truly love and admire her for all that, The person she is.
I'm so lucky to have had her in my life.

Pacific Coast Wonders

I have always had a hard time expressing what I want to say, what I feel. Writing has never been a way for me to express myself, except now. Why so much secrecy in my life? I've always felt tremendous amounts of pride, yet I was always very modest. The way I lived my life came naturally to me so I don't see anything I've done as special. Now I feel it's really important to stay Happy, Healthy and Honest (My 3 H's). Whatever <u>Happy</u> means to you.

I was at a beach far away from home, facing the Pacific Ocean in Oregon. There was a cool drizzle that early morning and I was dressed in layers, carrying a maroon cloth pouch, incense and matches. Inside the six- inch flowered pouch with pink drawstrings was a baggie with some of Christine's remaining ashes. Down the beach I saw people walking their dogs and I was afraid they'd trample on the ashes if I flung them into the wet air. I walked closer to the to the ocean's edge and watched the waves come toward me. The water was ice cold but that didn't seem to bother the seagulls. The bundled up couples and their dogs passed behind me. I was relieved I didn't have to say good morning or acknowledge their existence. The drizzle stopped and I sat on the wet sand, clutching the pouch. The summer flowers reminded me of another bright time at the beach five years earlier.

That morning had been sunny and hot in East Haven, Connecticut. Christine and I were going to the beach across the street from her apartment. Jason and Mika were on their way to see the new, animated Hercules movie with Andy. We packed salami and cheese sandwiches, peaches and iced tea. We carried sand chairs and *People* magazines. Christine picked her usual spot on the right near the water. There was a slight breeze coming from the south. We positioned the chairs so we'd face the sun. Our faces relaxed under dark sunglasses as our bodies molded into the chairs like the true sun goddesses that we were. Our big toes slowly dug into the hot dry sand at the same time.

"Ahh, Connie, there's nothing like the sun at the beach. If only we could just stay here always. I promise I'd never be bored, I'd never complain, never want for anything else."

"What about everybody else around us?" I asked. Not wanting to exclude the others and wondering how we would fare alone.

"They could come visit us here. You do mean the kids don't you? Everyone else can wait."

"Yeah, our kids, but what about the others?"

"It doesn't really matter. I just wish I could do my life over again. I'd be strong, smart, and happy. I'd leave for the west coast and settle there; that's where my heart really is. Maybe in another life I was a California girl."

"But you're already strong and smart. I don't know many people who have your strength to live alone, make decisions, live with pain. You've got more smarts than most people. Don't knock yourself," I said anxious to make Christine comfortable, if not happy. I wondered how I'd do if our positions were reversed. I was afraid I'd be weak and dumb, weak with self-pity and dumb with pain. I'd be unhappy too.

"I got no choice. This is IT for me. What am I going to do about it? Yeah, I've cried but then what? I'm still breathing even thought sometimes I wish I wasn't. I'm still fighting, so I guess I want to live some more whatever it takes. Breathing's a hard habit to break."

"Lots of people just give up. I'm afraid I might be one of them," I said.

"Nobody knows what they'll do 'til they're in it. I used to say, Shoot me if I get this far, if I look like death warmed over. Even better, call Dr. Kavorkian! Now, I look like shit, but I still want to live."

"You don't look like shit!" I shouted knowing she spoke the truth but not wanting to give in to it. Her face was a sunken mess; her body was mostly bones. Her black bathing suit hung loosely around her fallen breasts. God, how had this happened? Why had my sister gotten into such a mess?

"It's okay, you don't have to lie. I've got nothing left to look at in the mirror."

I looked over at her and wondered how she's made peace with this part of herself. I kept thinking it was something I could never have done. I'd be tempted to fight the ugly fight like my father, defying death and its power by saying, "I won't go willingly and I won't go quietly." A lot of good that had done him; he died alone. Alone was not how I wanted my sister to feel as long as she was still alive.

Wet and weary was how I now felt on the west coast beach that morning, three years after my sister's death. We were heading out to continue our travels up the coast. The trip so far had been wonderful. A week earlier my family and I had left Chicago for a ten- day vacation. We had landed in Sacramento on June 20, the anniversary of Christine's death. Back to my dear friend Bram's home; this time he'd agreed to drive the four of us north up the coast in his new blue Volvo. I wanted the kids and Michael to see the magnificent Redwoods, the ocean, the mountains and Mount St. Helens. Along the way we'd stopped to see my son's birthmother in Oregon, where we'd been staying in a large comfortable rented beach house.

Suddenly I wasn't sure I wanted to release Christine's ashes there. It was dark and gloomy. Maybe I should have done that in San Francisco when we visited days earlier, where Bram and Kermit took the kids and Michael on the cable cars while I slept in the car. But it was cloudy and windy there too and we hadn't been close enough to the water. On the ride down, I had developed a migraine headache that lasted all day. Nothing helped. At my old friends Jay and Brian's I couldn't eat or drink a thing for lunch without throwing it up. I felt terrible, but later couldn't help wondering if the migraine had had something to do with the heaviness of my memories.

I liked traveling with her ashes. Maybe I should just take them back home with me. It started to drizzle again and I held the flower pouch closer to my chest and wondered, What's the big deal? Most of her ashes were already scattered: in the Atlantic by Andy and Joan, by me and my family in Lake Michigan and some already in the Pacific farther down the coast by Tina. I'd saved a thumbnail's worth back home. I wanted a part of her with me, but I also wanted to make sure Christine had done her share of traveling. Suddenly my heart said, *Yes*, this was the right place.

I looked around and didn't see anyone, so I opened the pouch and pulled out the baggie of ashes. I took off my sandals and walked into the cold ocean. I stopped when my ankles were covered in white foam and unzipped the baggie. Seagulls came flying overhead looking for food. Several stopped and waited nearby. I looked inside at the dark mix and quickly turned the bag upside down. The ashes floated briefly into the air like suspended time and then scattered around my feet like dead ants. I was relieved they were in the water. I lighted seven sticks of incense and planted them in a circle in the wet sand behind me. The seagulls watched but didn't move any closer. I looked up at the clouds and said out loud, *"Christine, it's the ocean, the water you so longed for. Smell the salt, touch the wind, see the waves, hear these words, and know I will never forget you."*

Could she hear these words or were the words really for me? The salt, the wind and waves took away the ashes and I was left with an empty plastic bag. I bent down and filled it with wet sand and broken shells. The exchange didn't feel fair, but I clutched the heavier bag to my chest anyway. I walked back to the beach house to pack up and leave for the next part of our journey north.

Days later we were in Seattle at the movies. (We'd just arrived the day before at my girlfriend Janice's home to celebrate thirty years of friendship.) It was raining and we didn't know what else to do with the three kids after having eaten at Buca de Beppo's and walked through Pike Place, the oldest farmers market in the country where live fish are thrown across the room to startled passersby. Jason, Mika and Janice's daughter Lauren wanted to see "Scooby Do." Janice, Michael and I were going to see "My Big Fat Greek Wedding" next door. At first I hesitated, not sure I wanted to see a funny movie about Greeks.

"Come on, it'll be fun," Janice said.

"I'm just afraid it'll be full of stereotypes and I'll get mad," I said but also thinking if it was well done I might get mad anyway. Greeks have a knack for bringing out the worst in me.

"Michael says he'll go, how about it?"

The times worked with "Scooby Do, so I said, "Guess I'll give it a try."

"It's just a movie, no big deal," Michael said in his usual casual manner, as if to call attention to the way I can be excitable over nothing at times.

The movie made me cry. Oh yes, it was full of stereotypes but they were lovable ones I wasn't familiar with growing up. There was no mean anger, no threats of violence, no hatred. There was plenty of love and good humor. The dad was a comical restaurant owner who didn't hesitate to let you know the Greek origins of every word in the English language. The mom was large, energetic, and understanding. There was plenty of good food, lively talk and smiling people around. In the end the lovable thirty-year old woman Toula got to marry the lovable non-Greek, Ian, and they all lived happily ever after next door to her parents. This of course was after her non-Greek boyfriend agreed to convert to Greek Orthodoxy, marry in the Greek Church and do everything his in-laws wanted him to do.

143

An angry part of me thought, "Yeah, it's all right, as long as you agree to do what they want, but what if you've got a mind of your own? What if the non-Greek refused to convert? What if the girl refused to beg him to do it for her? No Greek Church wedding, no wedding at all. You'd hear them wailing and pulling the Greek girl off the handsome pagan." Naturally I was thinking of the time two decades earlier when it had happened to me, when Michael and I had married without his converting, without a Greek Church wedding, despite my parents' pleading with me to talk to him about it. I kept thinking, "the guys a Japanese Buddhist for God's sake. Why would I even think of asking him to convert?" I suppose the answer my parents had wanted to hear was that we'd do it for them; he'd make the switch for them, as if changing religions were as simple as changing sheets. Naturally I was also thinking of the time three decades earlier when Christine had been forced to marry a Greek guy she hadn't known. Where was the fun in that?

Another, quieter part of me watched as the happy dad kissed his daughter on her wedding day with pride. It was a moment Christine and I had never gotten from our father. (It's a moment I sometimes dream is happening now between my father and sister. Didn't she die on Father's Day so she could finally get that longed for kiss, that longed for pride a father must give to his daughter?) I suppose it was this acceptance into the folds of family love that made the movie sad. If only we could've been another kind of daughter – the kind in the movies, sweet and only slightly rebellious, nothing terribly serious that couldn't be worked out in the end.

We walked out of the show with most of the audience still laughing.

"I haven't laughed so hard in awhile," Janice said.

"It was better than I thought it was going to be," said Michael.

"Yeah, it's good as long as you agree to everything they want. Maybe you should have converted. Then maybe my dad would've smiled just like Mike Constantine." I said knowing nothing could've lightened my father's load of sorrow.

"Hey, it's only a movie!" he said, laughing as he put his arm around my shoulder. The kids were waiting for us in the lobby.

"Hey Mom, "Scooby Do" was fun! What took you so long? We've been waiting twenty minutes, let's go! Jason said.

"What was your movie about Mom?" Mika asked.

"Oh, it was about this girl who wanted to marry a guy who wasn't Greek but it all worked out and everybody was happy in the end." I said.

"It sounds interesting," Janice's daughter said. She was almost 14, a tall, blond beauty.

The six of us linked arms and walked out of the theatre into the warm rain. Our deep friendship wasn't something to be taken lightly. It wasn't something the movies could easily imitate. It wasn't something I'd ever take for granted.

Certainly I'd never know what my sister didn't take for granted. There were things I knew to be true, and there were things I would never know. I knew she had lived her life the best way she knew how. I knew she had struggled to stay alive many years past her expected demise. I knew she hadn't spent a lot of time complaining.

What I'd never know was how much of her spirit had been buried deep inside her heart, how much of her potential had been fulfilled, how much of her true essence she had allowed others to see. Naturally, in wondering about my sister, I have wondered about myself. I'd like to think my heart hasn't buried a great deal, that my potential hasn't gone untapped, that my true essence is visible to all those who take the time to look. But then I also think that no amount of unveiling will erase the truth that none of us wants to face, that one day we will all die. This computer I'm typing on may outlast me. This house may outlive us, certainly the trees outside will.

During our vacation we stood beside the giant Redwood trees thousands of years old and we stared up in wonder. How could something so huge live so long? How could trees live longer than humans? How could we understand the language of trees? The same questions could be asked about the Cascade Mountains, Mount St. Helens or the ocean itself.

On our way to visit the redwoods, Jason and Mika had wanted to see the famous redwood that Julia Butterfly Hill had lived in for two years in order to save it from destruction. She had won and wrote a book about it, a book Jason had Hill sign when she came to their school the previous year to speak.

On that trip, he had wanted to touch the tree, to look up and see where Julia slept and ate.

But Bram said, "We may not be able to go into that area; the lumber company owns it and they don't want trespassers on their land."

"I hate those lumber companies, I hate all the cut wood I see, I hate those big trucks that haul all the beautiful wood away!" Jason said.

"Hey, our picnic table is made out of redwood, lots of furniture is made out of it. It's long lasting and useful. We need to use the wood." Michael said.

"Not our table, I didn't know it was made out of redwood! It doesn't look red at all," Mika said.

"Well, I think we should close down all the lumber companies and save all the trees forever and ever." Jason cried. He had been a stick lover since the age of two. He had a collection in the backyard that he played with and guarded carefully. He adored climbing trees and could spend hours running back and forth along the pavement swinging a stick like an orchestra conductor. No one messed with his sticks.

Later, inside the Humboldt Redwoods State Park, Bram asked two volunteers about Julia's tree and they confirmed that the tree was on private land and that the condition of the redwood was uncertain. Rumors had it that the tree had been damaged or chopped down. The evils of the lumber company were discussed and we left knowing we wouldn't be able to show the kids Julia's tree. We continued our drive and stopped to tour a nearby lumber town despite Jason's protests.

"I don't want to see this stupid town. Evil people live here doing evil things, cutting down my redwoods!"

Mika was quiet looking around, and so was I. Bram and Michael talked about the people who needed to work in order to live and how we needed the wood to build things and how cutting trees wasn't bad if it was done right and other trees were planted. Nothing would ease Jason's outrage.

"I don't care what you say. They shouldn't be cutting down any of these trees."

I didn't know how many redwoods we really needed to cut down. I only knew it seemed tragic to cut so many down once they'd lived for hundreds and thousands of years. It seemed like they ought to be able to die a natural death and not have us interfere with the cycle.

I suppose I will always feel the same way about Christine's death. Her natural cycle was cut. Didn't nature mean for her to live to a ripe old age? I suppose I'll always feel that way whenever I hear of a life cut short. Was that really necessary? Did that person need to die at forty-seven or forty-three or thirty?

Soon after we got back home I read about the early death of a former neighbor named Sophia. She died of breast cancer at forty- seven, the same age my sister had been when she died. Her handsome Greek husband worked with Michael and they had both came to our wedding. Sophia was a beauty with long dark wavy hair, flawless skin and a gorgeous figure. I envied the ease with which she carried herself. She hadn't talked like a loud or embarrassing immigrant. She'd had class, something I hadn't, until then, seen in Greeks. In my younger years I'd felt awkward and unsure and had hidden it behind a tough exterior. I hadn't felt Greek or Macedonian or American.

I'd felt caught in the middle, the way I sometimes feel living in the Midwest instead of on either coast, where I sometimes long to be, as if living by the water's edge would better define who I was.

I learned of Sophia's death by reading the obituaries, something I never used to do but now almost enjoy. I read them like short biographies wanting to know how a life gets summed up. I'm usually disappointed and ask, Is that all they have to say about a life? What was that person like? How can someone's life get reduced to nothing?

I read Sophia's obituary quickly and was sad that there was no picture. It was long, about half a column. I learned that she had been the daughter of Greek immigrants who ran a restaurant in New York, that she had majored in art history, loved to cook and started a culinary school called Global Feast. Her husband was quoted, "She read cookbooks the way people read novels. To her, shopping for fruits and vegetables was not a chore; it was something she delighted in." I held the paper on my lap for a while, closed my eyes and imagined Sophia cooking with her two daughters in her warm kitchen filled with love. It was a satisfying eulogy. I was reminded of a *New York Times* collection of memorable obituaries in which the editor notes,

"When reading an obituary we've turned to the end of the book to see how it comes out. Death is the end of all that awesome potential that the infant brings into the world and each obituary is a tale about how well someone fulfilled it."

Sophia's story told her life's tale or at least some highlights from it. That was something I'd tried to do for Christine in her obituary, something we'd worked on together a year before her death. I remember bringing it up on the phone one morning.

"I don't care," she had said. "I'll be gone, I won't be seeing it. Say whatever you want."

"Why not think about it and write some stuff down. I could help you with it if you want." I said not believing I'd ever be having this conversation with my younger sister.

"How would I even start? I have no idea where to start and where to end. I'm not good with words like you are."

"It's not an easy thing for me either, but I could send you some examples. What about that? It's totally up to you," I said having no idea how I would begin or end either.

"Go ahead. No hurry though, I'm not planning on leaving anytime soon!" she said with a laugh.

"I've seen writing exercises that suggest writing your own obituary as an assignment. I'm in awe of people that can actually do it," I said.

"Sorry, I won't be around to help you with yours."

"That's all right. I'm not planning on leaving anytime soon either!" We both laughed and moments later we hung up the phone.

Is it fate that determines when we live and when we die? Do we really only have so much time allotted to us when we're born? If that's so- and sometimes I think it is- then do I want to know when that is for me? Would that help me to live a better life? I'd like to imagine packing up and moving to the ocean and watching the waves and heavens from my house high up on a mountaintop without a care in the world. Visitors would come to bring me their time, attention and love and then they would leave. I'd be left with my books and flowers, photographs and paintings and the world would spin happily in my direction, at least for a short while.

Christine had her short while. She lived for eight years with the virus knowing nothing is permanent, nothing is certain. She lived knowing she had a short while to visit the West, to kiss her grandchild, to drink iced tea on a hot summer's day and swear that was the best thing she had ever tasted. She lived a full life with each breath and that's all any of us could ever hope for:

Inhale life and Exhale love.

Afterword

It's the summer of 2003 and as this book goes to print Shag, Christine's dear cat has just died of old age. He had been living with Andy for the past four years and they were inseparable. Christine's grandson Mikey had open-heart surgery several years ago to fix a hole in it but now he's fine. Tina had a baby girl and she's named after her Yiayia Christine. Another baby is due on Thanksgiving; it's a boy. The youngest Kerry is moving ahead with her life after some setbacks. The oldest, Adriana is by all accounts well. Next Father's Day, on the fifth anniversary of Christine's death, my family and I will take part in painting a bench on the beach with the Artists on the Wall project. The stone benches overlook the pier where parts of Christine's spirit will always remain. Her work is complete. Life moves forward.

I'm finally doing what I always wanted, in a sense; I'm leaving here for good.